# Praise for *Winning The Mind Game*

"This is a very important book for the field of appl[...] must for any practitioner wanting to work effectively [...] Rowan's work starts where all other books leave off. [...] the clinician with some very powerful intervention tools and strategies for both problem solving and performance enhancement. If you're serious about developing an effective sport psychology practice, then *Winning The Mind Game* and it's techniques need to be a part of your clinical armamentarium.'
– **Dr. Alan Goldberg**, Sport Psychologist, author of *Sports Slump Busting and Playing Out Of Your Mind*, former #1 Tennis singles player and twice Conference Champion for the UMass Minutemen, former teaching professional

"The importance of sport psychology in training became apparent to me decades ago, before it was developed into an applied science, and before there were specific words to the different concepts. I have been incorporating it into my work since, and encourage the same of anybody working with athletes to enhance performance. *Winning the Mind Game* is a terrific tool for helping them do exactly that."
– **George H. Morris**, Silver Medalist, Showing Jumping, 1960 Rome Olympics, Prior co-Chef de Equip (coach) for the United States Olympic Show Jumping Team

"As a coach and counselor/therapist for over 20 years, I have used many of John's ideas for performance excellence, and have found them to work exceptionally well. This book truly synthesizes those ideas into an easy-to-use, comprehensive framework for all performers. My athletes, and clients, have responded powerfully to these techniques, and I highly recommend this book to anyone looking to 'win the mind game'."
– **Peter Thompson**, Head Swimming Coach/ Sport Psychology Instructor, Ursinus College, Collegeville, PA

"The active alert trance states that Edgette describes in this book are, in my view, essential to enhanced performance in competitive golf. As a psychologist and competitive golfer I have experienced first hand the dramatic improvements possible when an active alert trance state is induced and maintained."
– **Thomas H. Mallouk**, PhD, Clinical Psychologist, 3 Handicap Golfer

*"Winning the Mind Game* is a step-by-step guide for professionals who have a basic familiarity with hypnotherapy and want to expand their practice by working with athletes on performance enhancement. Edgette and Rowan offer a clearly written, welcome addition to the literature that provides information about building a sports performance practice from both the administrative and clinical perspectives. Highly recommended!"
– **Jeffrey K. Zeig**, PhD, Director, The Milton H. Erickson Foundation

# Winning The Mind Game

## Using Hypnosis in Sport Psychology

**John H. Edgette, PsyD
and
Tim Rowan, MSW**

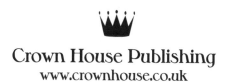

Crown House Publishing
www.crownhouse.co.uk

First published by

Crown House Publishing Ltd
Crown Buildings, Bancyfelin, Carmarthen, Wales, SA33 5ND, UK
**www.crownhouse.co.uk**

and

Crown House Publishing Ltd
P.O.Box 2223, Williston, VT 05495-2223, USA
**www.CHPUS.com**

**British Library of Cataloguing-in-Publication Data**
A catalogue entry for this book is available
from the British Library.

**ISBN 1904424023**

**LCCN 2003102135**

Printed and bound in the UK by
*Biddles Ltd*
*Guildford and King's Lynn*

## *Dedication*

To my little boy Austin, may you grow into a winning mind
to go with your winning body.

*John H. Edgette, PsyD*

Emmy, Vanessa, and Shera.

How could any one dad be so lucky! Thanks for being
so awesome and wonderful and for bringing such great
pleasure to my life!

*Tim Rowan, MSW*

# Contents

# Acknowledgments

My greatest thanks goes to the love of my life, my wife, who has taught me so much about sport psychology in her writings, lectures, clinical works and most of all as world class show jumper waiting for the horse.

Thanks to my friend and teacher, Jeff Zeig, who continues to pass along so brilliantly what he learned from Milton H. Erickson.

We remain greatly indebted to the Crown House US Sales Director, Mark Tracten, who has actually midwifed this book from start to finish. Without his support and encouragement, this book never would have happened. Helen Kinsey, Clare Jenkins, and Rosalie Williams at Crown House have all been a pure joy to work with. We have never worked with individuals that were so talented, professional yet so easy to work with. Together with Mark they truly seem to be a publishing best-case scenario.

Special thanks goes to students and associates, Joe Dowling and Patricia Peters for reading over the manuscript, seeing what I could no longer see and indexing it to boot.

My greatest thanks however goes to my wife's show jumping instructor, Olympic silver medalist and co-Chef de Equip (coach) of the Olympic Show Jumping Team, George Morris. As a young man, I lamented never being able to study sport psychology by closely watching Lombardi at work coaching his players. I have gotten even luckier. It has been a privilege to stand by the in gate next to you. I can only hope for more lessons ahead. May Jan find the horse you wish for her.

*John H. Edgette, PsyD*

Without Joe Rowan, my brother and assistant head coach in boys soccer at Bishop Walsh High School, none of the success and resultant championships would have been possible. Thank you!

A special note of thanks to other assistant coaches, Dr. Raul Felipa, Dr. David Searles, and Steve Wilkinson in boys soccer. Fred Tola and Amy Owens in girls soccer. Tiffini Wagner, David Karelis, Bill Devlin, John Groetzinger, and Jerry Rice in softball. I would also like to thank Jim Zamagias, Athletic Director at Bishop Walsh, for his support over the years.

A note of enduring appreciation and thanks to Brenda Mathews, colleague and secretary, for her help and expertise in clerical and computer services.

*Tim Rowan, MSW*

# *Introduction*

This book elucidates our ideas as practicing sport psychologists and clinicians who became greatly enamored with the ways in which current developments in Ericksonian clinical hypnosis could be used with athletes. After years of employing these state-of-the-art techniques with a wide range of amateur and professional sport clients, we realized the promise that hypnotic interventions held for the field of sport psychology. It became rapidly apparent that our work was very different from how other sport psychologists were practicing. Other sport psychologists, both academicians and clinicians, were mired in an unrelenting and redundant emphasis on visualization and relaxation. To the extent that they were using hypnosis, they would often be making direct suggestions for perfect performance ... "you will be stronger, you will run faster and faster each and every time you race," etc.

We began to recognize that we had developed a very special model of sport psychology that took full advantage of the current developments in the field of clinical hypnosis. The time was ripe for a book on hypnotic sport psychology that would teach clinicians already versed in hypnosis how to apply their skills to this new population. Although we both teach and offer workshops on this topic, we know of no book that deals with brief strategic and Ericksonian interventions in hypnotic sport psychology.

This book is written for the clinician who knows the basics of hypnosis but who is either not working with athletes yet or not working with them in these sophisticated ways. The reader will be taught assessment and intervention techniques with both adolescent and adult athletes at all levels of competition from serious recreational to professional. Both individual and team performance is addressed.

Many clinicians have been fascinated with sport psychology but have not known how to get started. They either have had few ideas about conceptualizing the problem and an appropriate treatment or intervention, or been handcuffed by traditional notions of imagery and relaxation. If they employ those techniques, they wind up feeling bored or ineffective and athletes often find the techniques superficial. This book provides specific strategies that will enable clinicians already using hypnosis to begin practicing sport psychology in a way that will be satisfying to them and to their clients. Therapists who are looking for ways to expand their private practices and see new clients will find this new population rather exciting. Athletes as patients are extremely dedicated to improving their performance and thus are open to techniques that may cause resistance from other clients. This book may very well create for you a new and exciting client base that will both challenge and reward you at the same time.

We hope you enjoy the read.

*John and Tim*

# I

## *Theoretical Considerations*

# Chapter One
# *What is Clinical Sport Psychology?*

The domain of clinical sport psychology is very broad. We define clinical sport psychology as helping athletes overcome a variety of psychological symptoms and problems. We also see the domain of the clinical sport psychologist as helping athletes to acquire certain psychological, cognitive, behavioral, and affective qualities, so that their physical capabilities are enhanced. So the province of clinical sport psychology not only includes the removal of that which hinders but also includes engendering psychological qualities that will help athletes to go even further in their quest.

This book focuses on helping the reader who has a basic knowledge of how to use hypnosis in therapy to begin applying those skills in working with athletes, and we describe a number of advanced hypnotic interventions to bring about this therapeutic effect. As in clinical work in general, however, hypnosis remains a tool, albeit an invaluable tool, to influence the subconscious mind quickly and effectively in order to promote change. After all, that is the clinical value of hypnosis: it enables change, often very difficult to achieve, to occur more quickly, easily, and effectively. Talk therapy with general clients or with athletes can sometimes, even often, be effective, but, for clients who have difficulty changing or those who want to change especially quickly (athletes can be most common among this group), hypnosis becomes an extremely useful catalyst.

Just as in general clinical work, where symptoms limit a person's ability to experience a full and satisfying life, symptoms limit athletes' ability to perform and win. The clinical sport psychologist also can help athletes adopt certain psychological qualities that help them to more easily achieve their potential. What separates clinical *sport* psychology from clinical psychology in general is that, with athletes, the goal is always improved performance on the playing field, wherever that might be. In general practice, people wish to overcome symptoms to make a part of their life more satisfying or to free them from psychological anguish or pain. In the field of clinical sport psychology, the goal is equally important in our opinion, and that is better performance and better results.

We do not agree with the sentiment that sport psychology is a separate field requiring extensive specialized training and a special set of credentials. We hold the opinion that any competent therapist with an extensive interest in sport can learn to adapt his or her strategies to working with this group, so long as the therapist is trained in current and cutting-edge brief therapy approaches. Athletes are even less interested than the everyday person in a long-winded telling of their life story in the service of developing insight. Competent and dedicated therapists with an interest in helping athletes can easily learn to work with this group. The issues that athletes face and the symptoms that they have are similar if not identical to those experienced by the general population. With the athlete, what the symptoms impact upon are her athletic performances and not her ability to give sales presentations, make love to her partner, or hold back her anger when disciplining children. The goal is always improved performance in the gym, on the field, or on the court.

We emphasize hypnosis in working with athletes because of its ability to create change quickly and effectively. It is a sophisticated tool that allows us a great deal of power and control in the service of our clients. This contrasts with the way in which we feel the field of sport psychology has sold itself horribly short: by a traditional emphasis on visualizing perfect performance and on achieving deep levels of relaxation. Later we will discuss how this is a gross oversimplification of what the athlete needs and is often totally irrelevant.

# The fifty greatest athletes of the twentieth century

A wonderful and interesting way in which we can best illustrate the full range of problems that face the athlete is to sample the issues that some of the world's greatest athletes have faced. Many of them were profiled in a turn-of-the-century weekly show offered by ESPN, the cable TV sports channel, entitled *SportsCentury: The Fifty Greatest Athletes of the Twentieth Century* and aired throughout 1999. Let's take a look at some of the psychological issues they faced and were able to overcome. This will give a very good indication of the sheer breadth of the symptoms, issues, and quandaries that athletes face. It illustrates how the traditional sport psychology notion of helping the athlete to become faster, stronger, and more perfect is an unnecessary attenuation of the focus of the field.

One baseball player who was profiled was Willie Mays. When Willie Mays first came up to the major leagues from the minor leagues he was a young man from a segregated small town, bewildered as well as insecure and immature. It was so bad, in fact, that the veteran African American player with whom he roomed tells the story of how at night Willie Mays would crawl into his bed and fall asleep in his arms for comfort. That's insecurity at a level seldom seen in the professional leagues and could probably only be talked about from the distance of time and in consideration of the greatness of Willie Mays. And ESPN points out that he started off his career hitting very poorly going one for twenty six. He thought about leaving the New York Giants and going back home and quitting baseball forever. But, fortunately, he had a manager who, like many great coaches, was instinctively an excellent sport psychologist. Leo Durocher sensed that the young man was trying too hard and was feeling dejected and said to him something to the effect, "Don't worry, son, just catch the ball and the rest of the team will hit for you." This intervention had the intended effect and he became one of the greatest hitters of all time.

Another athlete profiled on the ESPN show was Walter Payton. This mild-mannered and humble man was for many years the National Football League's leading all-time rusher. And yet, in the waning days of his career, he still had not won a Super Bowl ring. That was to change in his final year, when two of his hotshot and showboating teammates, quarterback Jim McMann and the overstuffed lineman turned running back, "The Fridge" William Perry, turned their team, the Chicago Bears, into a circus, albeit a winning one. They won the Super Bowl, but in so doing highlighted their own achievements and sent Perry into the end zone for a running touchdown instead of paying homage to their long-time great running back, Walter Payton, by giving him the ball and letting him score a Super Bowl touchdown. This decision by the coach Mike Ditka created a situation where Payton needed to deal with disappointment and player-team relations that were less than ideal and certainly not respectful. It is unknown whether Walter Payton ever did or would ever consider working with a sport psychologist to deal with such a situation, but nonetheless many others would—and this scenario certainly speaks for the breadth and depth of what the athlete needs to deal with. Traditional conceptions of what a sport psychologist could do to help an athlete are thus understandably shattered.

One of the greatest track and field stars of all times, Edwin Moses, had to battle numerous issues in his life, some external and some internal. First and foremost, early on in his career he had to persevere through a lack of environmental and contextual support for his capabilities. His high school not only didn't have a track team, but didn't even have a track! So he needed to look inside for hope and perseverance so he could continue until he found a place where he could realize his capabilities. Later on, during a world-record string of consecutive victories in the hurdles, he needed to find a way to maintain his focus and stay sharp while decimating the competition repeatedly. This he seemed to do again and again and yet, when he finally did get beaten, it was because he seemed to let up in the final stages of a race that he was leading, and an ardent opponent surprised him by charging past him just before the finish line. Over time, in the life of this great athlete, he had to deal with innumerable issues, all of which could have been addressed by a clinical sport psychologist. This one life nicely illustrates the range and the depth of the psychological needs the athlete has for psychological help.

Dealing with strong impulses usefully is a thread that runs throughout the ESPN profiles of many of the athletes. Alcohol, substance abuse, and sexual addictions abound. These people, the elite among athletes, often surmount these problems or achieve success in spite of them, and yet the world is full of athletes who do not fare as well. Those who seek the counsel of the sport psychologist will fare better. The great baseball player Mickey Mantle was shown in the ESPN program to have immense struggles with alcohol and with marital issues. He repeatedly said that, because no males in his family lived past forty, he never bothered to take care of himself physically. So he did not train hard but he did drink hard. And, while he remained married to his wife, Myrtle, he nonetheless spent much time with his mistress and publicist right to the end. Yet at the end he held a tearjerker of a press conference, at which he showed great remorse for the decisions that he had made and the weaknesses that he had, such that others could learn from his mistakes.

Edwin Moses wasn't the only great athlete who needed to navigate the choppy waters of media and fan relations. The great swimmer, Mark Spitz, is profiled in the ESPN program as being very unpopular and unable to keep the endorsements that he perhaps deserved due to what was said to be a rather unlikable personality. This was coupled with the immense public image debacle that took place when he left the 1972 Munich Olympics and returned to the US while the world was dealing with the Israeli athletes having been taken hostage and later murdered. This Jewish athlete was perhaps seen as self absorbed to focus on all the gold medals that he had won individually while his Jewish brothers were being murdered. Others speculate that his unpopularity was due to his waving his sneakers at the crowd while on the podium. Some saw this as a rude and insulting gesture while others felt it was a blatant shoe advertisement.

Dealing with fans and press is a thread that runs throughout the ESPN show. Ted Williams, for example, is revealed to be cantankerous and crotchety, rarely, if ever, speaking to the media. But he did show an incredible capacity to muster poise and to remain cool under pressure, as he became the last person to bat .400 in a baseball season. Ending the season over .400 was assured and yet he refused to not play in order to lock in that number but instead risked dropping below .400 by insisting on playing and having more at bats. On the last day of the season, his team, the Boston Red Sox, were playing a double-header. They wanted him to sit out both games and then, after he had played the first, they wanted him to sit out the second; but he refused, and wound up actually raising his batting average to .406.

However, the fact that the world's greatest athletes can navigate an issue or muster a much-needed quality doesn't mean that anyone or everyone else who needs to can do so without some assistance. As specialists in the psyche and in how to change it, we bring a unique set of capabilities to the table that deserve to be in the entourage of the athlete.

Like Mark Spitz, one of the all-time greatest pitchers, Sandy Kofax, also had to deal with issues involving religion and public relations. Though far from a devout Jew, Kofax nonetheless felt that he needed to be a good role model for Jewish youth and he refused to pitch the first game of the World Series because it fell on Yom Kippur. This created quite a controversy, which haunted him his whole life but was no doubt mitigated by the fact that he pitched the second, fifth and seventh games of the World Series with his usual awesome effectiveness. But this incident was far from the only psychological challenge Kofax had in his career, because in his youth he was not very effective as a pitcher. In fact, he was having so many difficulties that at the end of one baseball season, rather than put his uniform into the bin for washing ready for the next spring training, he threw it in the garbage can, intending to quit baseball. The trainer must have known that he would eventually have a change of heart because he fished it out of the garbage can and put it in the laundry bin. Only his tenacity and perseverance enabled him to come back and play some more, a move that eventually positioned him for glory.

Kofax was eventually helped by a catcher who discovered that he was trying to throw too hard. Becoming too effortful is one psychological problem many athletes have. And in many sports trying harder yields less. So the catcher encouraged him to throw less hard and to loosen his grip on the baseball. This resulted in the great success that he had throughout his career. And yet it wasn't just at the beginning of his career that he needed to deal with emotional and psychological issues. At the very end of his career, he also needed to decide whether or not to retire. He was at the height of his game and yet his arm was often so sore that he was told by his physician that if he continued pitching he may permanently lose use of it. So he decided to retire at an early age and at the peak of his performance, but not without great angst. Helping athletes to decide whether or not to retire and how to deal with being out of the limelight is a great contribution that clinical sport psychologists can offer. Of course, this issue takes an interesting twist for Kofax, because he is very shy and private by nature. He, unlike most others, does not struggle with what to do outside of the limelight but instead is criticized for not being a more active role model. He was so private, in fact, that, on numerous occasions when his residences have been discovered, he has moved to remain private and anonymous.

Pete Sampras was another one of the ESPN's fifty greatest athletes of the twentieth century. For a long time in the nineties he dominated the world of men's professional tennis. He was known for being cool and totally unemotional. Yet, during one big match, Sampras struggled to hold back tears. His long-time friend and coach, Tim Gullkinson, was dying of cancer. Sampras was so distraught by what was going on that he was having great difficulty focusing against his long-time nemesis, Jim Courier. As Sampras wiped away tears while being beaten, his friend Courier made the mistake of making a well-intentioned joke. He said, "You know, we can play this match some other time if you wish." And that had, for Courier, the unfortunate effect of refocusing Sampras, who went on to win that match.

This illustrates how still yet another aspect of everyday life can force the athlete to deal with personal issues that might encroach upon his or her game. The ESPN show also illustrated another frequent sport psychology need, that of discipline in living habits. While Sampras did not need to work with the sport psychologist on this issue, other athletes certainly could use help in this area. Sampras changed his lifestyle by way of a personal trainer who came over to his house and promptly opened up all of the cabinets and ripped out the junk food and promptly threw it in the trash. Pete Sampras adhered to the regime, but, unfortunately, so many athletes can't, and need the help of a sport psychologist, just as a diabetic may need the help of a psychologist to change lifestyle habits in order to control blood-sugar levels.

Some athletes need to contend with racial and ethnic issues, too. When ESPN profiled the great baseball player Jackie Robinson, for example, they pointed out how he was chosen to be the first African American athlete brought up to the majors because they felt that he was tough enough to take all that would be coming his way. Later, in the same sport, Hank Aaron would have to endure many death threats as he approached and surpassed Babe Ruth's home-run record. Yet these are just two famous athletes making history. Other athletes with other than white Anglo-Saxon backgrounds have often been subject to prejudice and aggression.

Sometimes, as in the case of Roger Maris, it can merely be a matter of being out of favor and disliked that makes you a scapegoat. Maris lost his hair through alopecia due to the stress of chasing Ruth's one-year home-run record, and he certainly was never quite the same again.

Moreover, we tend to think in terms of current racial and ethnic prejudices, but need to realize that these change and vary by time period and by culture. For example, the heavyweight boxer Rocky Marciano was subject to extreme prejudice and name calling not only because of his Italian heritage, but also because there was a bias against Catholics during the time he was fighting. Fortunately, he used that as motivation to improve and to win, as have many other boxers. But of course this is not to say that other boxers and other professionals don't break or waver under these assaults. If someone can handle these matters for himself, of course, he does not need a sport psychologist, but many do.

# Other professional athletes

Whereas the above examples are drawn from the hit ESPN show *SportsCentury*, the everyday professional athlete struggles with issues that are relevant to sport psychology intervention as well. One example is the one-time Atlanta Braves invincible closer Mark Wohlers. Wohlers became most hittable when he developed a wildness problem, which has come to be called Steve Blass disease, named after the first victim of this disorder and characterized by a sudden inability to throw accurately in a game. But, interestingly, Wohlers said that his struggles could be in large measure due to his sadness over his difficult divorce and a concern over his ailing mother. When professional athletes are so bravely candid, we get to see how everyday clinical issues can impact upon their achievement.

Anger and impulse-control difficulties plague so many athletes. Take, for example, Mike Tyson, who seems to alternate between inappropriate aggression and inappropriate sexual advances and keeps himself constantly in trouble with the law. Meanwhile, the potentially talented running back Lawrence Phillips bounces from team to team because he's constantly in trouble due to his volatile anger. The usually levelheaded quarterback Jim Everett was taunted by a provocative interviewer, Jim Rome, about being fragile physically and reluctant to get hit. When Rome called him Chris Evert on national TV, Jim Everett charged him and they wrestled around on the floor until they could be broken up.

Sometimes the tables are turned. A number of years ago at the All-Star game, Pete Rose, who was banned from baseball, was being interviewed and badgered by a reporter, Jim Gray. Without the assistance of a sport psychologist, Rose somehow dug deep and did the smart thing. While usually very hotheaded and volatile, he kept his cool and did not bite the bait, instead calmly saying that the personal questions regarding the ban were inappropriate given the occasion.

Helping athletes with alcohol and drug problems is an additional area where the sport psychologist, using hypnosis, can help. An entire book could be written about athletes struggling with these issues, but a notable example is that of Len Bias, who was chosen second in the National Basketball League (NBA) draft by the Boston Celtics only to overdose on cocaine that very night at a party.

It is not just the world's most famous athletes—nor merely a smattering of athletes over time—who have issues that could be addressed by a sport psychologist. At the time of this writing, a cursory review of the daily newspapers' sport sections revealed the following psychology-driven issues.

*USA Today*'s sport section from July 26, 2002, for example, has a lead article that discusses how parents might be hiring skills coaches for their budding star children but may be neglecting teaching them leadership, fun, and passion for sport. These three things are all psychological, behavioral, and interpersonal experiences that can be developed and influenced under the eye of a sport psychologist. Again, hypnosis is often an invaluable tool for reorchestrating the emotional, cognitive, and behavioral balance in an individual psyche as it relates to the world and a team.

The August 4, 2002, edition of the *Philadelphia Inquirer* sport section discusses New England Patriot's offensive coordinator, Charlie Weis, who was battling to get back into coaching having suffered severely from the side effects of abdominal surgery. This brilliant coach has been consigned to very short days in the training camp, in a motorized cart, and both his career and no doubt his life are at risk. He understands his obesity to be entirely psychogenic in nature, saying that he has tried all sorts of diets and all sorts of programs to no avail. He is quoted as saying that it's now or never in terms of creating lifestyle changes that will be pervasive and that he will sustain for a lifetime. "So this is a lifestyle decision. Never again am I sitting here having a prime rib and baked potato," he tells the *Inquirer*. We would be willing to bet that he did not include clinical hypnosis among his attempts at a remedy; nonetheless, this case illustrates the wide range of potential contributions that hypnosis in sport psychology can make in athletics.

In the July 25, 2002, sport section of *USA Today*, the cover story is about the mother of Rashidi Wheeler, who continues to struggle with depression and bereavement having lost her son to heat exhaustion one year earlier. Linda Will continues to reminisce, and misses her son, who starred for Northwestern University's football team. Sport psychology can be offered to the families of athletes for a variety of reasons and not just the athletes themselves.

The golfer, Phil Mickelson, in the March 23, 2002, sport section of the *Philadelphia Inquirer*, defends his go-for-broke style of play against his detractors. While critics want him to play more conservatively in the hopes that the world's number-two player will become a week-in and week-out challenge for Tiger Woods, Mickelson firmly defends his bold and aggressive game. "If I try to just hit fairways with irons and hit the middle of the greens, it's no fun," he tells the *Inquirer*. "Personally, to play my best golf, I need to play aggressive. I need to create shots. The bottom line is, I'm not going to change for anybody, because I am not going to have the enjoyment of the game taken away from me. Nor am I going to have my best game taken away from me." Here Mickelson defends not only what he sees as being essential to enjoying his sport and not burning out, but also the style of play that he believes makes his game as good as it is.

We don't know whether Phil Mickelson ever consulted a psychologist, but others who struggle with this issue and struggle to be as resolute as Mickelson should consider it. Mickelson ends his interview by saying, "I don't care if I ever win a major. I am not going to play this game without enjoyment, without the fun I have now. I believe if I am patient I will win my share of majors." The world is filled with burnt-out athletes who have soured from too much practicing and too much incessant focus on technical proficiency. There's a great need in sport to keep the fun in it—not consistently and at all times, but as a piece of the game.

Athletes often need to deal with issues related to aging and the potential or actual deterioration in their performance. Sometimes, staying sharp and competitive means changing your game strategy: for example, the fast pitcher who becomes a finesse pitcher later in his career when his velocity drops. Others stay competitive by beginning to focus more and more on proper sport nutrition or strength training. Others accomplish this by some method of managing their mind so that they do not feel old, such as by using the hypnotic phenomenon of dissociation, perhaps even if they don't know anything about hypnosis or dissociation! At the age of 32, Andre Agassi, for example, remained dominant on the tennis court through this very kind of mental trickery. He's quoted in the February 28, 2002 edition of the *Philadelphia Inquirer* as saying, "I don't feel old when I am on the court. I just feel old when I'm pulling the hairs out of my nose."

Sometimes heroes on the field get their sport psychology from the "sport psychologists" of everyday life. In the *Philadelphia Inquirer*'s sport section of February 5, 2002, the football Super Bowl hero, Adam Vinatieri, who kicked a winning field goal in the last second against heavily favored St. Louis Rams on behalf of the New England Patriots, is quoted as crediting his unflappable confidence to his grade school teacher. When Vinatieri was nine it seems he could barely read and couldn't spell. He was classified as having severe learning problems, and was put in special-education classes. His teacher helped him to develop a healthy self-esteem with encouragement and support, and making positive predictions for the future. "Mrs. Farrand was the first teacher that actually motivated me to do good things. A lot of kids who start off a little slow in life or have a certain learning disability, they are already straddling the fence post. You can go one of two different ways then. You can let that affect you the rest of your life and say I'll never make it. I'll never do anything. I'll never be good enough. Or with the right influences you can use that as a stepping stone and say I have achieved this with a handicap, so there's nothing I can't achieve."

The story goes on to discuss how special-education teacher, Marcy Farrand, continually created and then supported that attitude. But the emotional support and encouragement and predictions for the future weren't the only hypnosis-related techniques Vinatieri benefited from. He also used some positive visualization of the practice field rather than the jam-packed high-intensity Super Bowl arena. He told himself, "Pretend it's the middle of June and you're on a practice field by yourself." Of course, it was January, not June, and he wasn't there by himself.

There were seventy-two thousand people at the Louisiana Super Dome, but nonetheless his mental trickery worked and he stayed cool under pressure.

## Looking in the appointment book

So far we have taken a look at the world's greatest athletes, other professional athletes, and a cross-section from current events in sport. Yet these examples all come from the world of professional or collegiate sport. All involve top athletes. It is vitally important, however, to realize that amateur, recreational, child, and adult athletes at all levels can benefit from sport psychology. We have given these examples because they are some of the more extreme concerning well-known sports people. Yet, again, it's very important to note that not only aspiring professionals but the most mediocre yet serious everyday athletes can and do benefit from hypnotic sport psychology.

A look in our appointment books for the week we wrote this passage is most illustrative of this point. On Monday, an eighteen-year old equestrian consults in an effort to become more resilient, having repeatedly burst into tears and blown her rounds after her rather harsh trainer asked her if she wasn't tired of losing and said to her after her practice that she definitely didn't "have it".

Later that same day, a sixty-year-old golfer comes in as a last resort. He has decided that he is going to give up his beloved game of golf if he can't overcome the "yips" (jitters in the arms and hands that some golfers experience when they get nervous while putting). We will teach him how to do self-hypnosis and invoke catalepsy to help his hands to remain steady.

We have general practices, so our sport psychology clients are scattered here and there throughout our clinical day and week. Tuesday afternoon, a high school wrestler, who is well regarded by his coaches, consults us because he totally dominates the competition until the final period of a tournament championship match. Something "psychological" happens, he tells us over the phone while making the appointment, and he always manages to lose. Today there won't be any hypnosis but instead an in-depth assessment of what derails him.

That evening brings in a woman who had been advised by her psychiatrist to give up her beloved activity of showing dogs competitively after she has developed anxiety and fears after a vicious and unexpected bite. Like most competitive people, she is angry and annoyed at the callous advice that she has received ("as if it weren't the most important thing in my life"). She consults us in order to work through her post-traumatic stress disorder so she can go back to the joy of her life.

Wednesday brings in a coach for a double session. He has recently discovered from parents and school officials that many of the boys on his high school ice hockey team have been drinking heavily. This all came to a head when last weekend they were doing shots of 151-proof rum and one boy was taken to the hospital in an ambulance to have his stomach pumped. The fact that he almost died brought the issue to a head. The coach wants ideas on how to manage this and prevent further incidents.

In the middle of the day on Thursday a squash player comes in. She's been invited to compete in a number of top tournaments around the world, but must raise funds from sponsors to cover her expenses. She laments that she never expected to have to sell herself. She muses that she always focused on being a good enough player to get to this level and now is having difficulty engaging in an activity that she not only detests but is not very good at—sales. She requests hypnosis to help her to adjust her attitude so she can do what she now needs to do in order to have athletic potential realized.

On Friday a young collegiate drives halfway across the country to consult us about his ability to "finish" in soccer. Having missed an important shot in a key game, he has become reluctant to shoot and this problem has become worse and developed into a pattern of avoidance. He will receive deep and prolonged hypnosis so he can be repeatedly age-regressed to when he was able to shoot comfortably and successfully. That history of success, once recovered and revivified in hypnosis, will then be linked to associational cues to the present, so that these memories can invoke a sense of confidence, making him want the ball so he can shoot.

We have now illustrated psychological factors facing some of the world's greatest athletes as well as psychological factors impinging on other athletes. This survey gives a good illustration of the range of sport psychology issues that can be treated hypnotically.

Ericksonian brief clinical sport psychology proceeds in a similar fashion to Ericksonian hypnotherapy in treating clients. That is to say the approach one uses in brief strategic hypnotic therapy is very typical to what is used with the athlete. The main difference is that issues, attitudes, and traumas are resolved in service of better athletic performance. But then again that's not so different from everyday clinical practice, anyway. People change in order to accomplish a certain something, not just so they can change. For example, instead of resolving a fear of flying so that a newly promoted executive can perform on the job, a job that now requires more traveling, the sport psychologist resolves that same fear of flying so that the athlete can travel to competitions around the country. The reason for change for the athlete is different but there still is a reason to change.

Owing to a modern idea of the role of the sport psychologist —one made possible because of advances in brief strategic and solution focused therapy—our notion of what is required to be a sport psychologist departs from the mainstream. First and foremost, we believe it is important for the clinical sport psychologist to have a background in one or more methods of brief therapy. This book emphasizes how the tool of hypnosis can be adapted to the athlete but also has a strategic and solution focused flavor. That's not to say that other forms of brief therapy can't be useful with the athlete as well; they most certainly can.

A second important quality is to be thoroughly in love with sports. The effective clinical sport psychologist needs to be a fan of at least one sport and in great depth. But of course it's useful to be a sports aficionado in general and at many levels of the game. And it certainly does help if you were and are an athlete yourself.

This leads to another essential quality: extreme respect for athletes and what they do. The world in general and the psychotherapy world in particular is filled with people who "don't get it", and can't see the value or importance of what an athlete does. Therefore, they see what sport psychologists do and what athletes want as being peripheral and trivial. They marginalize the work of the sport psychologist and are disrespectful toward the athlete. It is the exact opposite of this attitude that makes the successful clinical sport psychologist so esteemed by his or her athlete patients.

This point of view, however, is controversial. There is much debate in the field over what credentials the sport psychologist should have. Some see the practice of sport psychology as requiring mastery of a specialized body of knowledge, requiring specialized training and requiring special credentials and certifications. We disagree, and believe therapists should be licensed and certified by their profession and not defined by the type of problem being solved or the population being served.

Nonetheless, you would benefit from familiarizing yourself with the various positions in the field, amply discussed in *Exploring Sport and Exercise Psychology* (Van Raalte and Brewer, 1996). We have found this to be probably the best general introduction to the field at large.

Less theoretical and more practical is Jack Lesyk's book *Developing Sport Psychology Within Your Clinical Practice: A Practical Guide for Mental Health Professionals* (Lesyk, 1998). For more information on sport psychology and hypnosis you are encouraged to read Donald Liggett's *Sport Hypnosis* (2000). Liggett's book takes a more traditional approach to hypnosis and sport psychology but should be required reading for everyone interested in the subject.

It is also important to consider belonging to the various relevant sport psychology associations and to go to their meetings. These organizations typically provide information regarding training and certification. Most of the major organizations and their contact information are listed in the resources at the end of the book.

However you define what you do as a therapist, we are sure you will find that both your hypnotic and Ericksonian brief therapy skills, developed, honed and applied as discussed in this book, will prove invaluable.

# Chapter Two
# *Myths and Misperceptions of Sport Psychology*

The public at large, athletes in particular, therapists in general, and even practicing sport psychologists suffer from holding a number of ideas about sport psychology that are patently in-accurate. Many of these ideas remain as unchallenged assumptions that have been passed down from generation to generation of sport psychologists. Others are still believed because they become convenient ways for unsophisticated professionals and the lay public to explain and understand something that is actually quite complex and sophisticated.

There was a professor of psychology with a particular theoretical bent who summarily dismissed every other school of therapy through a process of explaining in only a sentence or two what that school of therapy was about, and then adding another tag sentence that illustrated limitations. Sport psychology often suffers the same fate. It is understood—or rather misunderstood—through the vehicle of a few sentences, and thereafter either dismissed or its potential contributions grossly minimized.

One of the most predominant misconceptions about hypnotic sport psychology and sport psychology in general is that it is primarily about anxiety reduction. However, most athletes do not want to or need to experience deep relaxation prior to or during their athletic performance. Most athletes in fact value the experience of being on edge, psyched up, pumped up. Too often, the gross overemphasis on creating relaxation leads athletes to become concerned that they are going to come up flat. Many if not most athletes are more interested in learning how to channel and manage their anxiety or, better yet, how to perform in spite of it. For example, the great Olympic equestrian and (at the time of writing) the coach of the United States Olympic team, George

Morris (2002), recounts that prior to riding in the 1960 Olympics in Rome he went out during the morning of the event and surveyed the course and immediately and definitively decided he wanted no part of it! He told his coach that he wasn't going to ride. Bert DeNemethy, then coach of the Olympic team, insisted that he ride, and grabbed the bridle of the horse and physically made the pair go into the ring. George Morris and Rio exited the ring with a silver medal. Later asked how he ever managed to get around the course under such conditions, much less get a medal, he said that he used the "do or die" situation to force himself to rise to the occasion and ride his best. He then humbly, hesitantly and quietly noted in a matter-of-face way that "this is not always the case with riders, some crumble under the pressure" (Morris, 2002).

Probably the second most predominate misconception about hypnotic sport psychology is that it is vital to imagine a perfect performance. While this strategy can be useful for some athletes, in some situations, the gross overreliance on this single method sells the entire endeavor of hypnotic sport psychology short. Moreover, this imagining a perfect performance is most often accomplished through the vehicle of relaxation techniques, deep-breathing exercises, and visualizations. These methods constitute "hypnosis lite", whereas the hypnotic induction allows for an experience that is more like virtual reality. Moreover, most athletes benefit not from visualizing a best case scenario but by experiencing having a mental stance, or a process, or a strategy, that allows them to deal with the many personal and team glitches that arise during the course of any event.

Another misconception is that sport psychology necessarily involves an extended period of therapy. This probably stems the field's dominance by psychoanalytic and psychodynamic practitioners in its early days. Psychoanalytically oriented therapists felt that any problem, small, medium, or large, required an extended period of therapy. Nowadays, with an Ericksonian understanding of psychotherapy, we recognize that most small problems and many large ones can be ameliorated in a relatively short time. In some cases, with a motivated athlete with reasonable psychological resources, the therapy can take place in a single session, especially if the therapist is clever enough to hit the bull's eye with his or her interventions.

A related myth that is that the therapy will by necessity foster an overly dependent relationship between the therapist and the athlete that will later hinder the athlete in competition. Of course, if things are going incredibly well, the relationship won't be seen as a pain in the neck but will instead be seen as a necessary lucky charm that needs to be carried around at all times.

This is reminiscent of the situation that appeared to take place for Atlanta Braves pitcher John Smoltz when he was returning to competition after his performance suffered from mental factors. For each game that he pitched, he would have his sport psychologist sit in the stands with a red shirt. TV commentaries would invariably at some point in the game flash to a picture of the sport psychologist in the stands in the necessary attire (perhaps to be spotted more easily?). While that sport psychologist would have considered such a relationship absolutely necessary—and certainly one can't argue with John Smoltz's success in those years— a modern understanding would have you believe that it was anything but. Erickson understood that the magic was not in the therapist, not even in the techniques, but was instead *inside the client,* and the techniques and strategies are but keys that unlock the doors to successful performance in sport or in life. Erickson made himself unneeded as quickly as possible.

Another misunderstanding is that improving through therapy entails uncovering deep psychological issues that are remotely but definitely related to the sport or performance issue at hand. In reality this rarely turns out to be the case. Problems in sport can be —and most often are—related to numerous other factors, including poor training, the experience of a sport-related trauma, habits that lumber on like dinosaurs, and the lack of opportunity to approach one's self and one's sport from an optimal mental framework or stance. Fortunately, these factors can all be addressed through brief Ericksonian hypnotic therapy.

It was once thought that, in the event of surface symptoms caused by deep psychological issues, you need to plumb those depths in order to have an effect on a specific sport-psychological problem. Now, however, it is understood that deeper phenomena can be effectively addressed and transformed through quality work directly on a sport symptom.

Yet another misconception is that standardized protocols will solve particular problems, no matter who is experiencing them. This leads practitioners to ask a rash of questions such as "How do you treat someone with _____" (Fill in the blank with "nervousness", "fear", "choking", "a slump" or whatever.) There are some practitioners who believe that there exists in psychotherapy a five-, seven-, or ten-step format for treating just about anything; that there is some sage, guru, or magic formula that will do the trick. We think otherwise. In our model, an individual assessment of each problem is made and a new mental infrastructure, designed for success, is substituted for the one that was causing the problem in the first place.

While many people have thought that sport psychology is useful or available only to the professional athlete or the elite amateur, it is increasingly becoming understood that anyone at any level who is serious about improving can benefit. And as we know, hypnosis is a most important tool to have in your toolbox for effecting changes. Thankfully, in this increasingly sophisticated world, adult athletes and the parents of child athletes understand —often even better than coaches do—that a sport psychology consultation can be an important or even essential part of success in sports. In a forthcoming chapter we will also discuss the use of sport psychology hypnosis with teams—an application that previously was seldom utilized.

Sometimes, athletes have shied away from sport psychology because they worry that they might have to practice boring techniques over and over again before the effects of the interventions are felt. However, with the advent of Ericksonian sport psychology interventions, the techniques are powerful enough, charming enough, and effective enough to necessitate only a small amount of practice. Moreover, that practice is interesting and invigorating rather than mundane and tedious. For example, athletes can be taught to put themselves into a light trance prior to going to sleep at night, so they can review desired improvements and give their mind tacit permission to work these into all levels of the psyche through the course of the night.

In the tradition of Erickson, we like to make hypnotic sport psychology charming, appealing, and efficient. Whereas Lars Eric

Unestahl (Unestahl, Edgette and Edgette, 1986) promotes his developmental model of sport psychology but says that any athlete employing it needs to agree to take two years to master it (and of course during that time be content not being competitive in his or her sport), we can't imagine, no matter how effective that model, finding any athletes in our practice who would agree to such a constraint. Unestahl cites athletes, Nick Faldo for example, as having benefited from his well-researched program, but it is hard for us to imagine athletes having the commitment and the trust to engage in such a training process, especially given the brevity of most athletic careers.

Some therapists and athletes alike fear that working on changing the attitude, perspective, or approach of a particular athlete through sport psychology will be too superficial to be anything other than temporary. They fear that other deep psychological factors will rear their ugly heads and that the changes promoted in the consultation will be too brittle and fragile to withstand the tests of time, anxiety, and occasional misfortune. Fortunately for both the athlete and the field of sport psychology at large, the reverse is true. As things change in the mind of the athlete, other complimentary changes then begin to accrue. In addition, such changes become deeper and more resilient over time. The changes created in a sophisticated Ericksonian hypnotic model create further changes that modify old patterns and structures and result in a new adaptive stance, attitude, or approach.

A final misconception in this field is that the endeavor is a rather somber and serious undertaking. While this may be true of traditional sport psychology, it is thankfully not so in current approaches. Benefiting from the whimsy and humor of Milton Erickson, the newer approaches are likely to be fun. This approach applauds, for example, such interventions as the pitcher in the movie *Bull Durham*, who breaks out of a slump by wearing a garter belt and stockings under his uniform; or the athlete who tries to stay loose by incorporating the posthypnotic suggestion of carrying a rag doll in his right hip pocket; or the athlete who seeks to recapture her swagger by responding to the posthypnotic suggestion that she take a series of hip-hop dance lessons.

Erickson was the first to legitimize the use of humor as a thera-peutic intervention. We intend to extend this into the field of sport psychology.

# Chapter Three
# *Using Hypnotic Skills in Sport Psychology: A New Model*

As we have seen, the traditional model of clinical sport psychology is based on two primary interventions: having the athlete practice being relaxed while engaged in sports; and having that same athlete imagine performing perfectly. The problems and limitations of that approach have been dealt with; this chapter will describe what our new model entails and provide a step-by-step guide to its implementation. The chapter will also summarize the step-by-step approach to implementation, as well as reveal the various decisions that need to be made at different junctures in each and every case.

## *The four elements of the new model*

Our model consists of four elements:

1. The athlete, if need be, is taught how to develop a proper mental *stance* or psychological attitude toward performance.

2. The athlete, if appropriate, is taught various cognitive and psychological *skills* that can be brought to bear in any performance situation, as needed.

3. The athlete is taught *hypnosis* and perhaps self-hypnosis—again, if appropriate—to enhance performance (in lieu of imagining).

4. As needed, the athlete is assisted in accessing *resources* that he or she has lost touch with from the past.

# The step-by-step implementation

These four elements—stance, skill building, hypnosis, and re-source retrieval, or SSHR—are the foundation blocks of our approach. The SSHR model can be implemented step by step.

First, the clinician needs to get over certain disabling assumptions about sport psychology. These assumptions handicap the clinician in such a way as to dissuade him from even entering the field of sport psychology. The first assumption is that sport psychology is a highly-specialized field and anyone who doesn't have extensive training in it should not engage in it. It is this type of logic that made a lot of highly capable and talented clinicians unnecessarily abandon the field of substance and alcohol abuse and leave it to specialists. It also led capable clinicians who are fully adept at helping people with bereavement to abandon that area and refer clients to "grief counselors" instead. We believe well trained clinicians in most instances can apply their professional ability to the diagnosis and treatment of a multitude of problems.

It is important not to let yourself be intimidated by the athlete who is consulting you. This is a greater challenge when the athlete is a star in your favorite sport. Hero worship simply won't work when it comes to providing a useful clinical consultation to an athlete. Don't ask for autographs or tickets to games.

You may not realize that most athletes, when they go for a consul-tation, fear being used by the psychologist as an advertisement for their services. So don't ask for testimonials, and always assure the athlete that the consultation is confidential. Like clients whom you have helped to stop smoking with hypnosis, the athlete may at a later date, after being cured, boast to friends, family, and media that you and your hypnosis get the credit for the change. But that is entirely the athlete's choice.

If you do feel awed by the star client, you need to deal with it quickly so that you can get on with treatment. Use the resources that you have already cultivated as a clinician to accomplish that. By this we mean deal with these feelings as you would deal with clinical situations that you've already had. For example, handle them as you would when working with the CEO of a Fortune 500 company who, you speculate, could open innumerable doors for you.

As a practicing therapist, you have a long history of managing those issues so that they don't compromise therapy. A very similar process takes place for you when you are working with an athlete you admire. Rather than be intimidated, allow yourself to be more motivated. Don't try *too* hard. Remember also that the athlete comes to you not with her great expertise in her sport but with a problem or an issue that she has little or no expertise to solve. You do, and as such have every right to be the professional, the expert, and the one with the special knowledge, that allows you to sit face to face with any elite athlete.

In implementing the SSHR model you should also remain aware of the misconceptions we discussed in the first chapter, so that you don't inadvertently fall prey to them. If you do fall prey, your effectiveness might be severely compromised.

These steps to using the SSHR model highlight the fact that most of the barriers to practicing clinical sport psychology are psychological and cognitive rather than having anything to do with not having enough information or specialized skills.

Now that, as clinical sport psychologist, your "head" is in the right place, it is time to look at the practical issues. The next step involves doing an in-depth assessment of the athlete who is requesting services from you. This is covered in depth in Chapter Four. However, for now, know that the trick to doing the assessment with athletes is to think of their problem as you would any other symptom with any other client. People, athletes included, come to you wishing to overcome *something*. If you consider the athlete's need for change as being typical rather than as a specialized need that you know nothing about, then you will find that you can use what you already know in assessing and later treating her.

Having completed your assessment, you are ready for the next step, which entails developing your treatment plan. This plan should be replete with interventions appropriate for the requested change. At this juncture be sure not to fall into the trap—as a sort of easy way out—of creating of a deep relaxed state and then having the athlete imagine a perfect performance. Instead, assess on a case-by-case and highly individualized basis what is useful and needed. Often, hypnosis will be essential or at least highly useful. Two important classes of intervention include alert hypnosis (see Chapter Six) and developing certain hypnotic talents (see Chapter Seven). This may be a bit too much even for a seasoned therapist starting out in clinical sport psychology. As is always the case in doing therapy, it's hard to go from seeing no patients of a particular age group or who have a certain disorder to seeing lots of patients in such categories. So the next step involves bridging that gap and gaining a comfort level with athletes.

To this end, rookie clinical sport psychologists should find some volunteer, *pro bono*, or very low-fee clients to work with. These might be friends, children of friends, or acquaintances. They might also be amateurs who are strapped for funds or come from communities that are impoverished yet have athletes seeking to move up in their chosen sports.

Getting started doing sport psychology is the biggest and hardest step towards developing this specialty. By seeing lots of clients for free or for a low fee, you break the ice and begin to develop a confidence that will allow you to consider yourself "in the game".

The next step involves getting to know a great variety of sports and expanding the number of sports you are know-ledgeable about. Pick up the lingo and be familiar with current events. While this is easier in this day of ESPN, ESPN 2, and an array of other sport networks and specialty channels such as The Golf and The Racing Channel on cable, it still requires some effort.

Remember also that some of the athletes who most commonly consult sport psychologists belong to sports that are either less popular or receive less media attention. Here we are referring to gymnasts, figure skaters, and equestrians, for example. So often, other than in Olympic years, these sports don't get much coverage. Even so, you as a sport psychologist need to become a connoisseur of as many sports as possible.

Don't take this as a dictate, however—you can't know everything! When dealing with a sport that you are unfamiliar with or one that is relatively obscure, the most important thing is that you respectfully develop a deep understanding of exactly what is required of the athlete so she can perform that sport.

Remember also that athletes who practice rare or obscure sports understand that the average person is not going to be an expert. We have treated a number of athletes whose sport we have had little or no experience playing or even watching. We have been fortunate to treat them successfully by going to great lengths to understand exactly what it is they need to do to be successful in their sport, whether it is curling, dog trials, or chess.

Another ongoing endeavor for as long as you wish to practice this specialty is an attention to your marketing strategies. We have more of this in Chapter Eleven. For now, just know that, as was once true for your hypnosis practice, you need to get the word out about your sport speciality, so that people will call you for services. When you first started practicing hypnosis, it was a specialty that was compelling to people. They would show great curiosity with the end result and that made it easy for you to talk about and market it. Practicing sport psychology is at least equally interesting to people. Therefore, once you get the word out, whether it is through Yellow Pages ads or brochures or a website, a trickle will lead to a stream of patients.

You also need to assess how broad a practice you want to have. Here you consider the extent to which you want to be involved with coaches and coaching clinics. Some therapists are comfortable working only with individuals; others enjoy working primarily with coaches. You should also decide how much you want to work with entire teams. Another consideration is whether you will want to work with children as well as adults, or just adults? The answers to these questions depend in part upon how you've answered similar questions with regard to your general clinical practice: for "coach", for instance, read "teacher" or "medical doctor".

The issue of whether or not you want to work with teams might be answered by reflecting on whether you were comfortable and interested in working in the corporate world as a therapist. Did you enjoy going off-site? Or did being out of your office provoke anxiety?

Whether you wish to work with child athletes may depend on how you get along with child patients generally. Have you had sufficient background in developmental psychology? Are you comfortable interacting with children? Are you able to present ideas to them in ways that they can understand?

## Summary

- Become familiar with the four cornerstones of the SSHR model: stance, skill building, hypnosis, and resource retrieval.

- Don't think of clinical sport psychology as being a specialized field that you don't practice.

- Don't let working with athletes put you in awe or intimidate you.

- Be aware of the myths and misconceptions of sport psychology.

- Do an individualized clinical assessment with the athlete.

- Develop a treatment plan complete with an individualized and broad array of interventions.

- Find low-fee or no-fee clients to practice with.

- Follow sports in greater depth and do follow a greater array of sports.

- Market to athletes, coaches, and parents.

- Consider the extent to which you want to broaden your practice to include coaches, teams, and children.

# Case-by-case decision process

Now we will look at a step-by-step approach to an individual case and the decisions you need to make, followed by a further summary for quick reference.

First, someone initiates contact. This necessitates your deciding who should be included in the first session. The person who wants the change the most should definitely be included. The athlete who needs to perform needs to be included. Anyone else who is either a help or hindrance can also be included. Also anyone who has a lot of power to create the needed changes is very useful to have in the session.

Second, decide what interventions need to be made.

Third, decide at what level the interventions need to be made: the individual level, the coaching level, the family level, or the team level. Obviously if the key interventions need to be made to change something the coach is doing, you need to develop contact at that level. If the family needs to be the focus of intervention, then you need to begin doing family therapy. If the team needs to be addressed then you need to seek access to the team. Individual, team, family, or coach hypnosis are all options.

In working on an individual case the next decision that needs to be made is whether the athlete seeking services (assuming individual treatment) needs to recover inner resources, develop a different mental set (or, as we say, "stance"), or perhaps to overcome a trauma. If it is the first, then you would consider things such as age regression and hypnosis. If the second, then you might turn to self-hypnosis and alert hypnosis to inculcate that mental set. If it is the third consideration then you might want to consider hypnosis for post-traumatic stress disorder.

At this point, the therapist needs to decide whether the intervention is an *event* or a *process*. An event is a one-time experience that changes things forever. If the intervention can be an event, the clinician might consider one deep and long session of hypnosis. On the other hand, if the intervention is a process that is going to unfold over a period of time and would most likely involve some practice or a development and implementation of skills, this would require a series of sessions of varying length.

Also at this juncture the clinician needs to decide whether the athlete has to remember to do something or remember to experience something in the heat of play. If something needs to be remembered or experienced on cue, the clinician then should consider using posthypnotic suggestions to facilitate that association in a given moment.

Another consideration involves whether or not the clinician should teach self-hypnosis or make a hypnosis tape to give to the athlete to support the session work. Both self-hypnosis and having a tape makes the athlete more independent and fosters the idea that the therapy is not just something that happens in the clinician's office, but outside, on the practice field and the playing field.

A final consideration in the unfolding nature of treatment involves whether or not to consider follow-up or booster sessions at regular intervals once the therapy has come to a reasonable conclusion. That is, once the goals of therapy have been met, the clinician should decide whether or not to suggest future sessions at some point to ensure relapse prevention (or health promotion) and to maintain changes that have been created. This consideration will vary from client to client. In any event, we never consider the end of therapy to be necessarily the final contact. An open door is offered for any future issues or needs that arise.

## Summary

- Decide who should be included in the first session.

- Decide what interventions are indicated.

- Decide whether an intervention should be made at the individual, coaching, family, or team level—or all four.

- Decide whether the athlete seeking services at the individual level needs to retrieve resources, develop a different mental stance, or overcome a trauma.

- Decide whether the intervention is an event or a process.

- Decide whether the athlete needs to remember to do something or remember to experience something.

- Decide whether to teach self-hypnosis or make a hypnosis tape.

- Decide whether to do follow-up or booster sessions.

# II

*Clinical Interventions*

# Chapter Four
# *Assessment of the Psychological Needs of Athletes*

The assessment of the psychological needs of athletes can best and most easily be accomplished by asking a number of solution focused and strategic questions. In line with our repeated emphasis that sport psychology should not be considered a field totally apart from psychology in general, and psychotherapy in particular, you will notice that these questions are very similar to those that any therapist seeking to provide a short-term strategic or solution focused outcome would ask. We have broken these questions down into four different categories:

- goal-oriented questions
- solution focused questions
- resource-retrieval questions
- contextual-support questions

*Goal-oriented* questions are designed to elucidate the exact outcome that the athlete desires. The second series is *solution focused*, which are designed to understand the particulars of what is desired. Whereas often the goal-oriented questions will evoke a lot of information about the problem the athlete is having, the solution focused questions are designed to help the athlete come up with ways to obtain that which he/she wants. We call the third group of questions the *resource-retrieval* group. These questions are designed to discover psychological, attitudinal, behavioral resources that can be used to obtain the goal. The fourth group of questions make up the *contextual-support* group. These questions are designed to discern familial, team, contextual factors and resources that will support the attainment of the athlete's goal.

# Goal-oriented questions

1. What would you like to accomplish in the session today and in our consultations in general?

2. How would you like things to be different when we are done working together?

3. What would your ideal outcome be? Encourage a "video" description, i.e. as if the client were describing a movie script.

4. What would be a minimally satisfying outcome?

5. How important is it for you to achieve this goal?

6. What are your goals in general as an athlete apart from what you are trying to accomplish with your work with me?

The first two questions are similar in that they are both designed to get a clear sense of what the athlete needs to accomplish in the consultation. Generally, the second question needs to be asked only if the answer to the first question is vague or otherwise unsatisfactory. Sometimes when people are unclear about what they would like to accomplish, asking them how things will be different gets a clearer response. Both of these questions constitute an excellent start to the assessment process inasmuch as any brief therapy, sports-oriented or otherwise, should start with a crystal clear conception of what needs to be accomplished. There also needs to be a clear, concise agreement between client and psychologist that the goal(s) they are working toward is the same. Satisfying results can be obtained only when specific and tangible goals are agreed upon by both parties.

The third question is designed to discover what a best case scenario might be. It is very useful to have a sense of what the ultimate and perfect outcome would look like, as an important reference point. To this end, it's useful to get a "video" description of the ideal outcome. By this we mean getting the client to describe the ideal outcome as if he were writing a movie script: he would describe in great detail exactly what the scene looks like, what each person is doing, people's verbal and non verbal behavior, and all elements of the scene that could reasonably be reproduced.

The fourth question is designed to serve as a complement to the third question. Knowing what the best case scenario might be, it's also very useful as a reference point to understand what the minimally satisfying outcome might be. This provides a reference point for what is the lowest outcome to shoot for. This actually isn't such a bleak question. Athletes are actually quite cheerful in saying something to the effect of, "Well, if I could improve my performance in that area ten to twenty percent, it would make a huge difference in my game!"

The fifth question is designed to get a sense of how compelling the need for change is. There are changes that are optional, changes that would provide some enhancement to one's performance, and changes that are essential to continued participation in a sport. By asking the athlete how important it is that he achieve the goal of the sport psychology consultation, you get a clear sense of whether it is urgent or merely icing on the cake. If something is absolutely necessary the athlete will be highly motivated to achieve it (while, on the downside, he may be *too* effortful in trying to succeed). If an outcome is only modestly important to an athlete, then he may not be focused and serious enough about change and this casual attitude may compromise progress. On the upside, however, there won't be as much pressure on either the athlete or the sport psychologist to achieve excellent results quickly. This can sometimes allow things to change more easily.

The sixth goal-focused question is designed to develop an appreciation of where the athlete is in his career. This will allow the sport psychologist to put the consultation, and the work of the day, in a proper perspective. It's very useful in terms of understanding the whole athlete to understand whether his aspirations are to be a competent recreational athlete or whether he is seeking Olympic gold.

## *Solution focused questions*

1. On a scale of 1 to 100, what would 100 look like as a best case scenario for your outcome? What would a zero look like? What is the closest to 100 you have ever been? Describe what that looks like. On that same 1 to 100 scale, describe where you are right now. Please describe what 10 points higher would look like. (The above are all considered scaling questions.)

2. What makes things better?

3. What makes things worse?

4. The miracle question: if tonight while you sleep a miracle takes place, what would be the first clues in the morning that this had happened? How would you notice the miracle had taken place while you were asleep and how would others notice that you were different from before the miracle had happened?

The first questions above—grouped as Number 1—are the scaling questions, designed to quantify in a very specific way tiny gradations of change. When the client can describe and clearly visualize what levels of the solution might look like, it begins the process not only of assessment but also of change. Anything that is intentionally visualized will act as a lure to the subconscious mind and help the athlete to organize his resources in that direction. Change will coalesce around that outcome.

The second and third questions are designed to help the sport psychologist and the client understand the factors that either contribute to the problem or contribute to the solution. Note that the solution is not always the opposite of the problem, but can be a cessation of the problem. In any event, understanding the factors that make the problem worse and those that contribute to a solution can enable the athlete to do more of what works, less of what doesn't, and to try something different. So many times problems result when a person continues to do more of what is creating the problem. These questions burst them out of that rut.

The fourth solution focused question is the miracle question, which is designed to assist the athlete to project himself into an ideal future where he is able to perform in a manner compatible with a peak performance. In this situation, he is able to imagine a preferred outcome and begin to work toward a future with desired qualities and characteristics. After the miracle has taken place, he can come back to the present and begin to make small incremental changes toward the desired outcome. For example, "What would be a 10 per cent improvement toward the preferred outcome?" would be a logical place to start.

Whereas the goal-focused questions allow both client and therapist alike to understand clearly their reasons for being together, the solution focused questions begin to elucidate what some of the needed changes might be. They begin to elicit information that the sport psychologist can use in the hypnosis to foster change. Interestingly, however, the change often begins to take place as the client answers the questions, in as much as it forces him to begin to visualize the solutions. Having visualized possibilities for solutions, the mind naturally begins to move in that direction. This is a subtle but very important intervention. In brief solution focused therapy, the assessment itself often constitutes an intervention.

## *Resource-retrieval questions*

1. Tell me about times when you have been "in the zone" and everything is going perfectly.

2. Tell me about times when you have had a peak performance.

3. Is anything in particular holding you back, inhibiting you, or blocking you from obtaining this goal?

4. What prior experiences have you had with sport psychologists or sport psychology, either good ones or bad ones?

5. Tell me about times when you have been performing at the level that you wish to obtain now, even briefly.

6. Tell me about times when you have had problems similar to this and how you have overcome them.

7. What are your strengths as an athlete, both psychologically and physically?

8. Have you ever been hypnotized before and how did it work? What do you know about clinical hypnosis employed by a sport psychologist? Do you have a good imagination? Can you be suggestible if you wish to be?

9. What have you tried to do already to get rid of this problem? What have you tried to do to bring about a solution?

The first two questions are designed to help clients to describe the anatomy of their prior successes in achieving the level of performance that they want to see now. Asking these questions and having the client answer them will enable everyone to focus on how what needs to be accomplished today isn't something new but is the revival of something that has already been experienced.

With regard to the third question, the sport psychologist will need to ask a number of follow-ups to rule out the factors being asked about. In particular, the clinician is seeking to make sure that there have not been traumas with regard to the issue at hand or such things as severe character limitations, which would then need to become a focus of the therapy in order for the goal to be obtained. An obvious example would be that, if the person comes to you wanting help with "jitters in clutch situations", it would be relevant and most useful to know if he had once choked and then been resoundingly booed and run out of town by the hometown fans!

Question 4 is designed to help the clinician to understand what the client's expectations are of the consultation. Prior good experiences with sport psychology means that the client will have a very positive expectation, which can be capitalized on, whereas prior bad experiences need to be dealt with so that the client doesn't go into the consultation being pessimistic or even fearful.

Question 5 is designed to help clients to elucidate further and describe in detail prior experiences of success. One really can't ask enough about prior experiences of success because it gives clients hope and optimism by having them recognize that they have already done what they hope to do now.

Likewise, the sixth question is even more specific in helping a person not just to focus on times when he performed at the level he hopes to perform at now, but also times when he burst out of the problem. This question then is designed to focus the client in particular on the anatomy of prior solutions.

Question 7 is designed to elicit both physical and psychological strengths and resources that can be brought to bear on the problem. Too often, people have problems because they have not used their usual capabilities and talents on the endeavor at hand. They are disconnected from their strengths and resources and have not applied them to the problem. This question is designed to identify what assets can be brought to bear on the problem. Later, hypnosis can develop these resources and can point them squarely in the direction of the problem situation.

The group of questions at number 8 are designed to assess informally both attitude toward hypnosis and potential hypnotic capacity. These questions enable the clinician to dispel myths about hypnosis and then begin to discern just how responsive the client might be.

Question 9 is designed so that the therapist doesn't fall into the trap of trying to promote a solution or curative idea that has already been tried, to no avail. The therapist also must do more of what works, less of what doesn't, and, importantly, try something different. It would be a waste of time to sell to the client the idea of change tactics that have been unsuccessfully tried. It's best to do something that either has been tried and been shown to work or has yet to be tried.

## Contextual-support questions

1. Is there anyone who wants this change more than you do?

2. Who's your hero; who's your role model?

3. Do you have friends, families, and teammates who are supporting you in your athletic aspirations?

4. Do you know people who have the kind of problem you are having, and, if so, how did they overcome it?

The first question in this series is designed to assess whether the person is taking the consultation for herself or on behalf of another person. If someone else is more motivated for this change to happen than the client, then that person should be a part of the consultation. It is also difficult to help someone to change when she is changing for someone else and not for herself. So an alternative is to help the client find a goal that she herself wants to achieve. Alternately, she can find some motivation for herself to want this change as much as someone else does. Often the someone else is a parent or coach and, for better or for worse, that influence needs to be factored into any sport psychology consultation.

The second question in this group deals with heroes and role models. These are people who are part of the psychological context of the athlete. So often from the time that someone has been five, six, or seven she has had one or a series of heroes and role models in a sport. It can be either someone she has just seen on TV or someone she has observed on the field. By helping the client to identify again with her hero or role model, she might figure out the way in which her hero or role model would address the problem that she herself is having. Of course, the client can also be encouraged to adopt a new hero and role model who had the problem she is overcoming and then she can identify with that person and emulate that person's formula for success.

The third question is designed to assess the resources in the person's immediate social environment. When the client assesses the extent of her support from friends, family, and teammates, she can begin, along with the sport psychologist, to discover ways in which these people can contribute to a potential solution. It's important for athletes to recognize that they don't have to do it all themselves, that they can ask others for help to achieve their goals. It's questions like these that have led some post-graduate students to refer to this approach as being strength-focused therapy or resource-focused therapy.

The fourth question of this group is a variation of the hero and role-model question. However, it is a question that addresses the ways in which the everyday athlete either avoids having this problem or overcomes it when she does have it. While heroes and role models can offer best case scenarios for working through a sport psychology issue, it can be heartening and illuminating to understand how the everyday "Joe" or "Jane" deals with similar issues.

# Integrating assessment and intervention
## Case study

Here is a case study concerning Shera, a seventeen-year-old soccer star entering her senior year of high school. There wasn't a need to ask Shera about her goals as an athlete because she came so well prepared for our sport psychology session. She and her dad (TR) had already written out what it was that she was looking to accomplish. The sheet that she came to session with looked something like this:

**Shera's Game Plan**
- More patience when receiving ball before releasing (survey the field before passing, shooting, or taking on the opponent 1-1)
- More aggressive on 50/50 balls—face the opponent and attack with a low center of gravity
- Continue to play your game and just strike the ball solidly
- Practice mentally/physically 1-1 moves
- Continued proficiency in use of left foot for passing and shooting
- Continue to put self in a position where ball is likely to land – come to middle of goal or far post but not near post

> *Note that the first six goals involve aspects of her play that she seeks to improve. The last two goals are psychological capabilities that can be encouraged hypnotically, and may in fact support the first six goals.*

- Elicit peak performances of past and link to desired current and future performances
- Posthypnotic cue to elicit what has already been organized/ planned for peak performance

Here is the transcript of my session with Shera (TR, Tim in the transcript, is Shera's dad, her coach and the co-author of this book, and he was present during this consultation):

**John:** What about times in the past when you have been able to do these things? There have been some times when …

**Shera:** I was thinking that when we played Allegany [High School]. The whole team was just totally together that game. I mean, just everything was on. Everybody just knew where the ball was going to be and we just—I mean it just felt like everybody was on a higher level than the other team. We were just clicking, everything was working and there have been other games where we haven't been as up, but for that game we were just so pumped and ready to go and ready to play.

**John:** So the team influenced you, you felt a group…

**Shera:** When the team plays well, I feel that I do better because like … just me I can't—I'm not eleven people, you know: I can't do it all myself. I am part of the team and everyone was just together. I mean it was just like that was our best game of the whole season last year because we were just … everything was working, everyone was together and no fights happened or anything. We all were just together and it was great.

*Solution-focused questioning.*

**John:** And that was the game that won the city championship. Excellent. So one of the things I am wondering is how you could have that happen even if the team was a little bit flat. How you could have that happen for you?

**Shera:** Of course I do want that to happen. I think maybe just always going for the ball and never backing down, never giving up and trying to encourage my teammates to do better. If everybody was flat and down and no one really had that much energy, then I could yell a little bit of encouragement to them. That usually gets people pumped up and then, you know, try to lead by example to do something everyone else could also do.

*Searching for the needed mental stance for control over performance.*

**John:** How can you make that happen without waiting for it to happen but to be able to bring that forth when you need it?

**Shera:** I think I usually get pumped in the game whenever. Well, actually, it is probably a 50/50 ball, or something like I win it and I can go through it and I get it and I go around them and I just sprint to goal. That's when I am just totally pumped and…

**John:** So if it starts to happen then it kind of escalates for you? So what if we were to start that happening mentally even before the game so that you feel the surge before it even began to happen on the field.

**Shera:** That's the idea.

**John:** But it seems to me that a number of these goals involve things that you need to be mindful of. To sort of keep that in your head. That you're capable of all these things physically, right?

**Shera:** Right.

*Answers that suggest the interventions of self-hypnosis, age regression, and post-hypnotic suggestion.*

**John:** It is kind of like you need to have them in your head so that you can do them, rather than forgetting to do them.

**Shera:** Usually, I think there is something about what the team does before games. We write down on a chalkboard right before the game, write down everything that we want to do and then we do a mental prep and lay down and the coach talks to us and everybody … I think that really helps me keep it in my mind a lot and I'm just not so much thinking about it. I just know and I just do it because I have been thinking about it and usually before I go to sleep the night before a game I review it. And then, usually before the game, the team gets together, he [coach] goes outside and does some stuff and the captains all get together in the locker room and we turn the lights off and everybody just sits down and goes through their own individual game plan, what they want to do. We sit there for about five minutes or so and then everyone just gets up and is pumped, and pounding the lockers and stuff and then we run out. It's more of a pre-game that we do on our own without our coach. But it is because of what he has told us that we know to do that.

**John:** Right, but there are still, you know, maybe five or six things here that you are capable of doing physically that you would like to do more regularly to move your game up. So it's kind of as if you need something in addition to all of that that will make this happen more consistently. I want you to learn how to use a cue to accomplish this. Then you can use the cue and you will automatically do what you have planned.

**Tim:** One of the things that I was concerned about was that I did the mental prep the night before the game and then they did their own pre-game. But if she gets flat or the team gets flat, you can't call timeout and talk to her, so you have to have some way to bring about a change while the game is taking place. And that is where your idea comes into mind and what we have already put down, which is some cue that brings this back to make it happen on its own.

**John:** So it is as if this is happening. You want more control. If it is happening naturally its happening. If it's happening as a result of the team's mental preparation, that's great. But you want a way to make it happen when it's not happening.

**Shera:** Yes.

> *Solution focused question searching for reference experiences from the past.*

**John:** Can you tell me about a time when the team was flat and you elevated your game in these ways?

**Shera:** I think I know: maybe Northern Bedford when I was a sophomore. We were playing up at Northern Bedford and we were losing 2–0 at half-time and everyone was kind of, you know, feeling down. A lot of people had given up basically at halftime; we were losing 2–0, it's hard to come back from that. But we were, I think, going uphill the first half. It was just a slight uphill—not straight up—so the second half we were going downhill. Our coach, my dad, made a prediction that we would come back and win 4–2, and we did. What happened was we were going downhill and I remember that I scored two goals, and then it got tied and everyone was pumped and everybody was going. After the first goal, I think everyone was kind of like, "We are back in it now, we can get it." So I mean that was definitely a time. I thought I was able to bring them out.

> *A prediction in sport is a natural use of age progression.*

> *More searching for what creates success.*

**John:** Do you remember how you did that? What did you think to yourself?

**Shera:** Well, I really didn't have much confidence at half-time, either. You hate to be defeated like before the game is over. We were just kind of down until he said we would come back and win 4–2. I was kind of, like, "OK, yeah, we're going to do it." I knew I had to score because, well, I just had to do it; I have to get everybody going. I remember that after I did score one of my teammates came up to me and said, "I knew that if anybody could, you could get us back into it." And that really, like, snapped my mind. Other people saw it, too. That's why I want to be the leader and everything.

> *Identifying a resource to bring forth hypnosis more fully.*

**John:** It sounds like determination is a good resource for you.

**Shera:** Yeah.

**John:** It sounds like also you can feed off things other people said. Like Tim predicts you're going to win 4-2, you can use that to really make yourself believe.

**Shera:** I guess I hate to say I lost faith. I guess I kind of did. Whenever he said that, I thought, I believed we can do it. Everyone had to believe in themselves.

> *Rapidly instilling hope via hypnotic age regression will be useful to her.*

**John:** Yeah, sure. Well, you know what would be really neat is if maybe we can move that internally so that you have that source of encouragement inside of yourself, if it wasn't in the environment. So, you know, you can bring it up, pull it up on demand. That way you are not really dependent on any enthusiasm outside of you. If it's there, great: you can feed off of it. But otherwise you'd have places to go inside of yourself where it will be waiting for you and you can tap into it.

**Shera:** That would be good because sometimes you know you can't count on other people to say the right thing.

**John:** Right, we'll do that. I think that will be a very good idea. Has anyone hypnotized you before?

**Shera:** Yes, my Dad [TR].

**John:** For what?

**Shera:** Pretty much, probably soccer or any other sport-related things.

**John:** How did it go? Did you like being hypnotized?

**Shera:** Yeah, it's OK. I usually, like, drift off, maybe sleep or something and then I don't know what he says sometimes.

**John:** So you kind of go into a…

**Shera:** … and then I wake up and its twenty minutes later, and I'm OK.

**Tim:** Probably the best example I can think of where this became important is that Shera was struggling at the beginning of last season and she wasn't scoring at the level that she was used to and I really felt that it was mostly a psychological problem. And so I said to her what we need to do is that we need to do something special here today and you and I need to go and work on this, just me and you instead of with the team. So I went through and really worked on helping her remember peak experiences from the past and then linked them to her desired outcome for the rest of the season. And she went from the first probably six or seven games with about eight goals—no seven goals—then she hit on a streak and she ended up with twenty goals in the last thirteen games. She had three hat-tricks in a row; one was a five-goal game and, once we got that going, she was back to herself. So I was able to use an individual session with her, actually at home, to set that up; and then we started, just her and I, we go out every night after practice and work on striking the ball solidly. So what worked was the hypnosis session as well as the deployment of a tactile cue. We went to the field near home and that seemed to reawaken her and then she got her confidence back and once she got her confidence, the season went fine.

*History of use of posthypnotic suggestion.*

**John:** Did you step up?

**Shera:** Yes, I remember that.

*Cultivating positive expectation.*

**Tim:** And Vanessa* [sister] has had the same experience. Even the softball team has done the same thing so they both have a similar experience. The softball team goes through the same process and they have been part of that.

**John:** So maybe one of the things that we can do today is help you to develop the inner hypnotist inside of yourself so that you can begin to do this for yourself.

*A new goal is to help her to become more autonomous.*

**Tim:** John, that is really my goal because I am happy with what I am doing but I really want her to be in a position so that she

---

*Vanessa sat in to observe since she was a psychology major at Mount Saint Mary's College in Emmitsburg, Maryland.

becomes her own resource and I am just icing on the cake that she can do this during a game if she needs it.

**John:** Right. Either that or we need to develop a special potion so that we can shrink you into the size of Jiminy Cricket and as she runs around the field you can be on her shoulder whispering into her ear. [To Shera:] Do you know any professional soccer players that you admire that do this kind of thing?

> *Seeding positive hallucination.*

**Shera:** Yes, actually, I read two books, one by Michelle Ackers and one by Mia Ham. They both talk about how you know that you have to be mentally there and you can't let yourself drift off to other things. You really have to be intense and stay in the game. And especially Michelle Ackers, because she has chronic fatigue syndrome. I think she probably shouldn't be playing soccer at the level she performs. She has to have so much inside of herself, like mentally, that she can just keep going and pushing herself. Like beyond, I guess, the point of exhaustion so after the game she's had, like, IV's put in her and all sorts of good stuff because she just has the drive to keep going and never giving up. She'll collapse on the field, go in the locker room, get an IV put in her and come right back out and play again. That is just, like, wow! I know that I don't have fatigue syndrome or anything but I couldn't imagine going through all that and still be at the level of play she has.

**John:** In the books do they talk about how they did it?

**Shera:** I don't think they really went into that. I can't remember right now but I don't think they went into detail. It's just like the mental game; it's like the names of the chapters that they talk about it, basically just say...

**John:** So they do this, and so you'd like to learn a way for you to be able to do it, too. Granted, you don't have chronic fatigue syndrome but that is just an extreme example of something someone needs to overcome.

**Shera:** Yeah.

**Tim:** And to piggyback on today, we're going to see Mia Ham play tomorrow. We're driving on to Washington but this would really be like everything that we did today could be affirmed even more by watching the best of the best, which is Mia Ham,

> *Seeding use of posthypnotic suggestion.*

play tomorrow and that would enhance all the stuff that we do. And then watching the other professionals play will be like an ideal performance that can become part of the posthypnotic work that we do.

**John:** Good.

**Shera:** Actually, one of the things in Mia Ham's book that really … Actually it's a quote by Anson Dorance (he's the head women's soccer coach for North Carolina, and he was the national team coach for a while). There is one quote that he said that she had in her book and I have heard before. It has something to do with the vision of a true champion. It is someone bent over, drenched in sweat, at the point of exhaustion when no one is watching. It is like how much that it takes out of you mentally to be able to keep going when no one is around. You could stop, no one would know, but you have to keep pushing on. I think of that when I am running and no one is around. I could stop, they would not know, no one would know, but me, but you have to keep going. Mentally, you have to just push yourself.

**John:** Right.

**Shera:** I really like that quote.

**John:** So, that is like something inside, it is pride. You are the only one that will know.

**Shera:** So, yeah, I ran five miles today.

**John:** Right. I think that one difference between a champion and someone who never achieves that status is that, rather than cutting corners when they can, they press on.

**Shera:** We run campus laps and some people cut across the baseball field, but you're supposed to go around the backstop. No one is out there watching you. It's whether you decide your going to do it or whether you decide you're just going to take a little break. And a lot of people run where the coaches can see them and then they start to walk and they walk around until they can see them again and then they run. And that really gets on my nerves. It's usually the young girls or something and I'll go by and I'll ask them if they are alright. I'll be like, "Are you OK?" and they're like, "Yeah, I'm fine." "Well, then, let's go, you know, let's run. You know you should try to push on."

**John:** It's universal. That has been the case forever. When I played football, I noticed that some people press just as hard or harder when the coach isn't watching. It's easy…

**Shera:** They sprint when they can see them. Maybe he knows, maybe he doesn't, but you know no one is going to tell on them. No one is going to rat them out but you can tell maybe later on in practice or in games who actually did it.

**John:** Absolutely.

**Shera:** I will say to them, "It's going to hurt you and if you don't do it it's going to hurt the team." If you don't do it bad things can only happen.

**John:** Let me ask you, now you know that you—that it is good to do these things and often you do them, [whether] you would like to do them more often. What stops you from doing them? You know you should do them consciously. When you are not doing them, what's stopping you from doing them?

**Shera:** What stops me with the 50/50 balls is the fear of getting hurt. You know you're coming at people and if you get hit there is always that chance, you know, that you're going to hurt yourself. I try to go through it most of the time. Ninety per cent of the time you're not going to get hurt. It's when you turn your back like I do at times that you do get hurt. So I try to tell myself just to go through it, that you got less of a chance to get hurt if you just go through it, but then, you know, you think, what if? And that is when you just stop and then you don't go through it. The last part, basically I just …

**John:** So that is the case with the 50/50 balls, a fear of getting hurt, but what about with the other things you wish to change? What stops you from changing with regard to those?

**Shera:** Well, probably the left foot. Obviously, I'm not afraid to kick it with my left foot, but it's not as strong. I want to get power with it like I have with my right, but it's just if I kick it with my left it will just dribble off at times. If I kick it with my right it goes nice and solid straight toward the goal. So I usually try to keep it so I'm shooting with my right, but if it happens to be my left I'm going to do my best. I guess I don't want to … I guess maybe it's not wanting to fail with my left foot and mess everyone up. I continue to put myself in a position where the ball is likely to land. I guess that's just something that I have to work on in practice. I don't know, maybe I have a tendency to go toward the ball. Maybe when the ball is coming downfield, I want to get to it first instead of waiting for someone else to get it to me. I really have to pretty much practice the one-on-one moves to do them in a game. It is not like you can't do them. You just have to practice them and you know sometimes doing OK but sometimes not. You might not do it OK in the game so it would just seem better to just not do them. I guess I just have to practice that more and get it perfected.

**Tim:** What about off-season skills training and camp this summer to get some additional coaching from the coach at Frostburg State University? She's already worked with Shera on the one-on-one moves and that is something that I think is very important for her game if she wants to continue past the high school to the collegiate level. She has to have moves and of course what she's just said is part of the problem. She wants to keep repeating the ones she's used to, which are OK, and some have been helpful to her, but the ones she is learning are more advanced. They are so different from what she has been doing she doesn't do them because they don't feel comfortable.

In order for her to feel comfortable she's going to have to practice on her own fifteen to twenty minutes a day just on one-on-one moves, separate from everything else. So that in a game this just becomes an automatic part of her repertoire. She needs to do it mentally first and then practice it physically on the field so it just comes to her automatically during a game. The coach told me the other day—I talked to her on the phone—that Shera's foot skills have dramatically increased. So it's coming, but she has to take the special time separate from other practice and do it on her own. It's got to be a discipline thing. I think it is more of a disciplinary task for her in the next couple of weeks as we get ready for the season.

**Shera:** Yeah.

**John:** OK, what else would be good for me to know in order to help you?

**Shera:** Well, I guess I can do all of these things, it's just a matter of, like, whether I practice them enough in my mind and on the field to do them. I just have to. I mean, I know I can do all this stuff with probably no problem. I just have to stick with it and not get down on myself or give up. I do that. I have had the tendency before to, you know, get down on myself and that's not good. I do that a lot, you know. I'll get angry with myself and say, "Why did you do that?" Then I'll kick the ground or something and that's definitely not one of the best things to do to try to get people pumped and stuff. A better idea would be to lead from the front since I'm a striker. Just keep my head up at all times and just, you know, if something bad happens, just let it go and move on and continue to play my game because I know I can do it.

**John:** From what you are saying, it sounds to me as if it would be useful for you to have a sense of trust and confidence that you can do these things, that you will improve at these things and that they are worth doing. Like practicing the one-on-one moves. If you believe that it will make a difference and you are going to get better at it, you'll do that practice. If you believe that using your left foot will be good enough—not as good as your right foot, but needed—and you can't favor your right foot too much or else it will limit your game, you'll give yourself an opportunity to kick more with your left foot and then that will improve in time, it will snowball. With confidence and trust in striking the ball solidly, but not super hard, you can choose to do something that's not your forte. So it sounds as if you need to believe in yourself a little bit more, accept what you are good at and then use this as the foundation to elevate your game where you need to improve.

**Tim:** Along the way up [to Philadelphia] we were talking about the concept that "less is more". Shera is reading a book on sport psychology entitled, Body, Mind and Sport. There is something that we need to take a look at and incorporate it and they have the idea that less is more. In golf when you really try to hit the ball hard, you get the muscles all tight the more you try to hit it hard and the less distance it goes. When you relax and are trustful, and just let your body do what it needs to do and let go, you end up hitting the ball much farther and hopefully straighter. So that is what she needs to do.

**John:** One of my sons loves baseball and he's a really good hitter and then he tries to hit a home run and he swings too hard and it pulls his body up and he winds up dribbling a little grounder for an out.

**Tim:** That's the idea: that if she could just relax and believe in herself. The last thing I would like to ask you, John, is that somehow we turn something around that could be a big deal in the back of her mind. Offensive Player of the Year as a freshman, Player of the Year as a sophomore, Player of the Year as a junior and so anything less than Player of the Year as a senior would be a letdown. How can we take advantage of and use as a resource state what she has already accomplished, as opposed to its being a deficit or an overwhelming expectation?

**Shera:** A little bit of pressure?

**John:** Yeah!

*The following is a highly individualized, conversational induction of hypnosis. The Ericksonian technique of utilization is demonstrated throughout.*

**Tim:** I have sensed that there was a little bit of pressure to do this again. Instead of something that puts pressure on her, how can we turn it into an inspiration? So we use it to our advantage as opposed to it being something in the back of her head that nags at her.

**John:** Close your eyes. I am sure that this is going to be a little bit like how it is when Tim hypnotizes you, but it will also feel a little bit different because, while we have a couple of things, a number of things in common, we also do things

> *Beginning induction by increasing curiosity with the presupposition that she will go into hypnosis.*

differently. So I think you will enjoy noticing that, while there are some commonalities, you will be able to experience some things that are new also, in a different style. Just as there are many ways and many styles of players in a sport like soccer, there's a lot of different but complementary styles of hypnosis.

So, Shera, as you allow yourself to listen to the sound of my voice, you can recognize that your conscious mind can focus on the things that I am saying, while your subconscious mind allows yourself to be influ-

> *Induction using conscious-subconscious dissociative statements.*

enced in ways that are right for you. So your conscious mind can assess and evaluate, while your subconscious mind can respond and experience. Your conscious mind can process the things that I am saying while your subconscious mind begins to actualize the things that I am saying. So there can be two complementary parts of you: part of you analyzing, assessing, thinking; a part of you reacting, experiencing, performing, implementing. And later on you may discover that this very same complementary way of living in the world is not only something that can take place in a hypnotic session, but is also something that can serve you quite nicely on the soccer field.

Now I don't know what kind of induction that your dad does with you; you certainly are welcome to hear his voice in your mind during a hypnotic induction, while you hear my voice outside of you,

> *Age regression and possible hallucination.*

suggesting certain things. So you can allow yourself to respond to the living memory. Of course, a memory once accessed becomes part of the present—indistinguishable from the present—so that you can respond to the memory of what your dad has said to you that's allowed you to relax so deeply at other times or you can respond to the things that I am saying now. So there can be a double-induction of sorts: something from inside helping you to go way deep down; something from outside also helping you to go down into trance.

It can be [that] you go into trance with every breath that you take a little bit deeper, one-hundredth or more deeper into trance, every breath that you take. While it might be

> *Induction and use of induction to attain the goals of the session.*

that with every word that I say you go one-tenth more deeply into trance. You don't need to try, because the harder you try the harder it gets. You are discovering, and you knew this, you're discovering the experience of effortless responding. And what you discover, here and now, will become a prototype for what you discover there and then, while you are playing soccer. As you go more deeply down into hypnosis, you can recognize that the fact that you have experienced hypnosis before means that can you have a certain inner confidence that you can experience it and respond again now.

Because you have already been Player of the Year there's pressure because you know you can do it. And isn't it true that you can look forward to this year, knowing that, because you've been Player of the Year before, it's something that is most doable,

> *Reframing to reduce pressure and anxiety.*

so that you can relax and enjoy knowing that you've accomplished that a number of times and that there is nothing that you need to prove; there is nothing that you need to do. Rather than being the exception, it is some-thing that is known to be possible from history. So, you can enjoy allow-ing your capabilities and skills to unfold.

Now I know that you want to face the opponent and attack with a low center of gravity on 50/50 balls. And you've had some fear about getting hurt, and that is understandable; but I would also like you to recognize that you've overcome the fear of getting hurt on numerous other occasions. You might go back in time to when you first learned to head the ball, and that certainly is an experience that most kids shy away from out of fear of getting

> *Age regression for resource retrieval.*

hurt. It's not so natural. And how is it that young kids get comfortable doing that or allowing the ball to hit them in blocking it, trusting that this is something that is safe, even though we may not feel that it is?

Now it's not a matter of fear, but it is counterintuitive to not use your hands. As a little girl, your first temptation was to catch the ball with your hands and you learned to never do that, unless you were playing keeper. So there's a lot of things in sports, there's a lot of things in soccer, that feel wrong, that are alright and you learn to do them. Being aggressive,

> *More age regression for resource retrieval.*

facing your opponent, attacking, low center of gravity, is just the next in a series of counterintuitive things that you have learned to do. But it's like that in many sports: you ride a horse, you want to hold on, you get a little scared, you learn not to squeeze with your legs because that makes them go faster. In baseball, it doesn't feel quite natural at first to put your hands on the bat the correct way; usually kids reverse it, because that feels natural and then you learn to do things the right way and it works out well.

| *Confidence-building through age regression.* |
|:---:|

You're going to learn that you have a wonderful opportunity ahead of you, to clearly move your game to that next level and to advance significantly. It can be the matter of some debate as to whether trust follows confidence, or confidence follows trust. It can be a matter of some debate as to whether first you perform well and then you have confidence and trust, or you have confidence and trust and then you perform well. You can avoid that, or recognize it, that you have a long history in soccer and in other sports; you have a long history of acquiring new skills and moving forward in your game.

This isn't the first time that you have done some things new: it's just the most recent in a long series of transformational experiences in your style and in your way of playing that allow you to get better and better. Years from now it will be something else, and you'll do that also.

Long ago, many, many years ago, you learned to ride a bike and it seemed so impossible at first, when the training wheels came off, to

| *Engendering gentle curiosity instead of debilitating intentionally.* |
|:---:|

balance on two pieces of rubber wheels and roll forward really quickly while moving your legs up and down, holding a little piece of metal in your hands so that you can go in the correct direction, hoping that you'd remember how to brake. It seemed so impossible, and yet you knew that other kids could do it so you gave it a try and you learned, and it worked. Later, perhaps, you learned to perform some tricks on your bike to go really, really fast. Sure, you fell; sure, you got hurt sometimes; but that didn't deter you. There's an inner confidence that you can tap into; you can trust in the wisdom of your body.

You know the only thing that is going to limit you is your physical capability and you don't know where that is yet and that's not your decision to make—that's not a limit that you decide. That's something that you find out and you don't know where that is and one day you will, but until then you keep giving yourself a chance to prove to yourself just how much you can do and how capable you are. Please don't let your modesty restrict you from finding out just how well you can play. And you can coach yourself with regard to this and all the other things that you need to do, need to know.

You've been blessed with a great coach; you've been blessed with great teammates. Now you have the opportunity of also—you haven't yet needed to, but now it's time—to discover that you can be your own great coach. You can be your own teammate so that when it's not coming from outside you can generate it from inside. You listen to that tiny inner voice. Perhaps you remember the movie *Pinocchio* and what Jiminy Cricket said to Pinocchio, when Pinocchio needed to develop a conscience in order to become a real boy. Jiminy Cricket said to him, "Conscience is a wee voice inside that you choose to listen to instead of ignore."

You've had good teammates, you've had a terrific coach, and you haven't needed to listen so much to that inner voice until now. It's going to be a great complement to what you have outside. When I first learned to

> *Positive auditory hallucination for achievement of session goals.*

meditate a wise Indian teacher said that we should experience 200 per cent of life: 100 per cent inner and 100 per cent outer. You're discovering that as an athlete. It's a natural part of a transforma-

> *Use of heroes and role models as an intervention.*

tion as you move from child to adult, from girl to woman. You also learn that you have more inside than you realized and you begin to look inside and draw upon that.

I have a friend who, when on the golf course, he goes inside and he beats himself up. When he goes inside he's very hard on himself. Yet he wants to become more like Jack Nicklaus and he says that, if you watch Jack play, he hits a bad shot, he shakes his head and says, "Oh, Jack" in an encouraging, paternal way. Knowing he can do better, supporting himself, not beating himself up. So Nicklaus became a role model he began to emulate.

It's time to take some risks; it's time to do some things that you know that you need to do rather than staying in your comfort zone. You can discover how much more there is to bring forth but unless you take that chance and use your left foot more and trust that you don't need to really kick the ball hard. You can go with what you're good at, what your talents are, play your game, develop your game and your skills and capabilities. It's a choice; it's a risk you're ready for now. And you can believe in yourself enough to give yourself a chance to practice it both mentally and physically, as a vote of confidence in yourself. You don't have to, but you want to. You can hear encouraging voices inside of you.

*Reinforcing suggestions for positive hallucination.*

You can reminisce back in time to times when you would bring forth your best game, your "A" game, or you can hear your dad's voice outside of you or your teammates' voices outside of you. And you can learn to do the same thing with a different team, even when the old voices are no longer there. Memory, once accessed, retrieved, recovered, reintroduced is real in the present. It's no longer the past; you can hear from inside, you can hear from outside, even when it's something that you choose to imagine.

You can pretend anything and it can be true. Wherever you go, you can shrink your dad and he can ride around on your shoulders. It can bring a smile to your face as you imagine him hanging onto an earlobe, clutching onto a collar; you make a sudden turn, he almost falls off; he's hanging on by one hand swirling around, just like Jiminy Cricket.

*Seeding what she will one day need to do on her college team, positive kinesthetic and visual hallucinations.*

My wife only gets to ride with the Olympic coach every couple of months, so, when she is off on her own, it's very important for her to have a way of believing that she can do the impossible. If you doubt it, it becomes impossible, as "impossible" as hitting a 90-plus m.p.h. baseball, with a little stick of wood. As "impossible" as kicking an inflated piece of rubber into a tiny corner of a net where it can't be deflected. As "impossible" as throwing another inflated piece of rubber through a metal hoop ten feet in the air from fifteen to twenty feet away.

*Encouraging self-trust, cautioning against doubt.*

Most things in sports are "impossible", like jumping a horse over four-and-a-half-foot fences. So it's very important at those moments that you close your eyes for a second. It doesn't need to be long. Remember doing it before, and remember the sounds of the coach's voice—and your dad has a very distinct voice, just as does the coach of the United States Equestrian Team. When you hear it in your head, it's like hearing it from outside. And the mind does not know the difference, you can know that.

*Maintaining awareness even while trusting self.*

You can think while you play, you can remain aware of what it is that you want to do, whether it is having more poise so that you perhaps pass or take on the opponent one on one or pass backwards or shoot. You can have poise that you access. You can think of where your position is and you can stay where you need to stay rather than where you are tempted to go. But that, too—I want you to remember that you've learned all of these things a long time ago in various ways.

When you were two, when you were three, when you were four, I don't know how old you were when you were first learning to play soccer. One of the first things you needed to learn was not to swarm around the ball. You see these little kids play and they are like a bunch of bees all swarming around the ball and one of the first things that you learned was to be in a position, stay in a certain place and not just go to the ball. Now it's time to learn some other things about where to be, where your position should be.

You know a lot more, Shera, than you know that you know, so I would like you to recognize that the things that you are about to do are very much like things that you've learned to do before. You have had a long history of success that you can draw upon. I don't want your wonderful quality of modesty to get out of control. And you should have a way of bringing all of this to mind any time you would like. So I would like you to pick a symbol of the work we have done here today—a symbol that will bring all of my suggestions right back to you, all of the other suggestions that would be useful right back to you from your dad, from other people, from teammates, from every source you can. There's a lot of coaches, and there's a lot of sport psychologists. I would like you to have a way of cueing yourself so that all of this is attached to some symbol. What would you like it to be? The sound of a whistle can come back to you, but you don't have the whistle, so maybe something else. The sweatband I saw in a photo your dad showed me would be a possibility if it is OK with you.

Everything can be connected to that symbol. It can immediately re-empower all of these suggestions. Maybe it will be touching your sweatband on your forehead, maybe it will be squeezing your left hand with your right—whatever you choose, it will immediately bring to mind all of these things and you will execute them with precision. Your mind will work in the ways that we have prescribed; your body will work in the ways that we have suggested.

*Ending hypnosis.*

So, with this in mind, you can allow yourself to take a couple of deep breaths and you can begin to bring yourself out of the hypnosis. Waking up all over, ready to discover how all of these things begin to manifest inside of you, unleashed with the help of the tool of hypnosis. Helping you to do what it is that you want to do, that you didn't know that you could do; your subconscious mind being free to assist your conscious mind. It's going to get a lot of assists this year, your subconscious mind, to your conscious mind, to your body.

## *Follow-up*

At the end of her senior season, Shera repeated as Player of the Year for the third consecutive year. She ended her high school soccer career as the Area's All-Time Scoring Champion with 97 goals and 33 assists for 227 total points.

# Chapter Five
# *Special Considerations in Inducing Hypnosis in the Athlete*

## *Hypnosis as the on ramp into "the zone"*

Most, if not all, athletes know what it feels like to be in "the zone". This is a state characterized by a feeling of slow motion, invincibility, incredible confidence, and a personal and experiential feeling of control. It is the state that athletes invariably describe as being present when they are performing at their best. For example, the year he hit 406, the Hall of Fame Baseball Player Ted Williams described the ball coming toward the plate as looking as if it were a beach ball moving in slow motion. Many pitchers in baseball are easy to spot when they are in the zone. David Cone, Greg Maddox, Curt Schilling, Randy Johnson, and Roger Clemens all make it obvious to the viewer that they are in a special state, and this can clearly be seen by looking at their eyes. They all look as if they have tunnel vision, and are relaxed but focused while being oblivious of their surroundings.

Now the importance of this discussion isn't just to highlight the characteristics of being in the zone or how athletes perform at their best when they are in it. The point is that, when hypnosis is successfully induced, it results in a state of mind that is similar to, if not identical, to being in the zone. The beauty of this news is that through the vehicle of the hypnotic induction the sport psychologist and the athlete get an opportunity to control entrance into the zone. Without the use of hypnosis, athletes have to rely on ritual and mood in the hope of entering into that sometimes elusive state. Some athletes get there more easily than others, but it is important to note that for our purposes hypnotic induction allows most athletes to enter into the zone regularly and predictably.

To help athletes see that hypnosis and self-hypnosis can accomplish this, it's important for them to recognize that the hypnotic state is not a passive experience. Too often, in our field of clinical hypnosis, people associate being hypnotized with sitting or lying down with their eyes closed, being very inactive and receiving the hypnotist's suggestions without doing much themselves. Too many people, hypnotists included, think that this is all hypnosis can be. This notion is at best a myth and at worst horribly limiting. Through the experience of active hypnosis, which can also be called alert hypnosis, the subject learns that hypnosis can take place even while he is active and interactive. To this end we provide specific protocols for teaching the athlete alert hypnosis such that they learn to go into trance while his eyes are open, while he is talking, and even while he is walking or running. The specifics of how to accomplish this are discussed in the next chapter.

It's important to educate the athlete that neither sounds nor sights need to be seen as an interference, a distraction, barring the way to successful hypnotic experiences. So a quiet room without distractions is not essential. The athlete and the practitioner should know that anything that can be accomplished in hypnosis in the optimal environment can also, with some work, be accomplished in any environment.

Educating athletes both about possibilities inherent in alert hypnosis and about being able to achieve these hypnotic feats in a noisy or visually distracting environment is of utmost importance to helping them incorporate hypnotic opportunities into practice and their performances. If the athlete believes that they need quiet or an armchair, then this self-limiting belief will be true. Being educated about the possibilities of alert trance and trance under any circumstances allows the athlete to discover just how much can happen in the arena. Without knowing that something is possible, however, it does not become possible.

# Age regression for hypnotic induction

One excellent way to drive home the point to athletes that hypnotic induction can easily put them in the zone is to use their prior experiences of being in the zone to create hypnotic induction! Milton Erickson taught that you could induce trance in a subject by regressing him back in time to various times when he was previously hypnotized. For subjects who do not have an experience in formal hypnosis, he would have them go back in time and re-experience times when they were particularly relaxed. These times might be considered normal everyday trance states. Now, of course, those strategies could be employed with athletes, but, since they no doubt have some experiences of being in the zone, if you regress them and have them re-experience those moments, then they will not only slip into a zonelike state but into hypnosis as well. It is important that the hypnotherapist suggest that they "go back in time and visit one or more experiences of being locked into the zone"; and then, as the client begins to do that, continually make the experience alive, vivid, and sensory. Then absorb the subject in these sensory experiences ever more deeply to strengthen hypnosis.

This induces the subject into hypnosis not only because he is revivifying historical analogs to the hypnotic experience, but because the very act of experiencing any hypnotic phenomenon tends to create or deepen trance. Thus deploying age regression as a hypnotic phenomenon serves a dual purpose. For more on using hypnotic phenomena with athletes, see Chapter Seven.

# Using the language of the athlete

In his never-ceasing efforts to individualize the hypnotic work to maximize its effectiveness, Milton Erickson always incorporated the specific language of the patient into his hypnotic pattern. So, to an accountant, he might say that they could "*figure* out a way of going down into trance" or suggest that she "*count* your way down into the hypnotic state"; to an engineer he might suggest that he "*design* a mental state that affords the opportunity to relax." In this tradition it is considered good form to use the language of the sport of the athlete to accomplish the hypnosis. This allows the athlete an extra measure of comfort and a feeling of familiarity with the experiences taking place. When a new experience is palatable to subjects, they respond more readily.

Examples of using the athlete's language to induce trance might be as follows:

- To a basketball player, the sport psychologist practicing hypnosis might suggest that "going down into trance can allow you to *rebound* from any fatigue ... and as you *pass* from one state of consciousness down more deeply into another ... you can discover that the hypnotic induction that you are experiencing can be an ideal *assist* to you ..."

- To a soccer player, the therapist might say, "You can allow yourself to effectively *block out* any unwanted interferences into your *territory* ... and when you want to and need to you can discover that you can *drop back* down into hypnosis ... and can learn to easily and comfortably use your *head* to *pass* down into trance as well as to *score* a certain comfortable physical experience...and you can discover that, just as offense can give way to defense and defense to offense as needed, you can have an effectively *overlapping* experience of being aware consciously while developing your subconscious resources ..."

- To an American football player, the language induction might be as follows: "You can allow yourself to move into an optimal mental *stance* ...and you can in hypnosis learn how to more effectively *tackle* a problem...this can *play* out and be *executed* exactly how we've been *practicing* it ... the deepening hypnotic experience can be like a time-out that you use to *rest*, *refresh*, and *strategize* about what is to come ..."

You will see from those examples how using the language of the athlete can facilitate a more successful trance experience. Hypnotic induction in particular can be accomplished more easily with this kind of individualizing and tailoring. The examples also highlight the need for successful sport psychologists to have some working familiarity with the athlete's sport.

# *The utility of rapid and brief trance experiences*

Owing to the requirements of sport, athletes need, often at a moment's notice, to access the hypnotic state, and get what they need from it. To this end it becomes very useful to teach the athlete how to go into hypnosis quickly and how likewise to terminate hypnosis quickly, or at least reduce the hypnotic experience to an optimal time period.

To develop this capacity it's beneficial to create one or more associational cues or triggers that allow the athlete instantaneously to go down into trance. It is helpful for these keys, shortcuts, or associational cues to be something that the athlete can either choose to do or not to do while also being something that is in his immediate surroundings during a sporting event. Thus, an athlete can condition himself with posthypnotic suggestions to go into an optimal level of trance (or the zone) upon touching the chalk, upon putting on his cap or helmet, or upon looking at his cleats. It is just important that the triggers be available when needed. If the athlete wishes to have this experience regularly and regardless of circumstance, the trigger can be something that invariably accompanies the athletic performance and inevitably will be present and contacted. If the experience is sometimes desired and sometimes not, then the cue can be something that is available but can be chosen, and is not necessary or essential. To create the associational cue the athlete should be told repeatedly in trance that the cue will elicit as much of the needed trance or zone or mental state as would be desirable in the given circumstance. Of course, key strategic interventions can also be set to come back upon use of the associational cue or trigger.

When a hypnotic state or moving into the zone is what is being triggered, the hypnotist should give the directive to go only as deep as is optimal, and remain in the state for only as long as required. For example, the night before a big game, while trying to get to sleep, the athlete may desire a very deep and stuporous level of trance. On the other hand, while planning a strategy to win the game, he may want only a light level of trance. Once in the zone, the athlete can learn to do whatever is needed. An example of this would be gaining confidence. Christian Latener, in the National Collegiate Athletic Association (NCAA) quarterfinals, when being called upon to make the game-winning (or game-losing) final shot, put himself into a zonelike reverie and had himself review times in his life when he had made just such a shot. This instilled a sense of optimism and confidence that allowed him to make the shot. Going into the zone is invaluable; athletes who experience hypnosis can then decide what to do cognitively and behaviorally while in the zone.

## Considerations surrounding induction and self-hypnosis

The question sometimes arises as to whether you use a hypnotic induction that can later be remembered and utilized by the athlete for self-hypnosis, or if you use a standard induction and simply make an intervention. The answer depends entirely upon what needs to be accomplished. If the athlete has as a goal accomplishing something that is predicated upon having an optimal mental state or stance, then teaching him self-hypnosis so that he can re-experience and recreate that stance is important. On the other hand, and particularly if the athlete can go into deep hypnosis, if there's a single habit or tendency that needs to be changed, once and for all, putting the athlete into trance and making strategic and suggestive interventions for change can be entirely sufficient. Since the athlete does not need to enter into a particular mental state, or a zone that will allow certain processes to unfold on the playing field, but instead desires a certain abrupt change in some aspect of his game, then more of a "one and done" hypnotic intervention can be used. When in doubt, however, choose an induction strategy that can later be used by the athlete to create a self-hypnotic state. This then makes the hypnotic tool the athlete's very own, and, even if the specific and focused intervention is entirely successful in session, later, if the athlete desires to make other changes or if he relapses, he can once again accomplish his goal.

# Chapter Six
## *Alert Hypnosis*

We have seen how the hypnotic state does not have to be a passive one for the hypnotized person. We know this from trancelike experiences in everyday life, such as driving hypnosis, where we might be taking a long drive to a familiar destination and eventually arrive without remembering any of the details of the trip. Throughout the journey, of course, you had to make left turns, right turns, stop, start, adjust speed, and pass cars, but all the while you are lost in a dissociated reverie. This is an excellent example of an eyes open alert hypnotic experience.

To work with hypnosis in such a way is a great aid to the athlete. This is true because when athletes receive hypnosis in the more passive fashion, it's harder for them to integrate into their play. Athletes need to be able to put themselves in a hypnotic state intermittently throughout a game or an event. Moreover, it's often helpful for them to perform their athletic endeavor while in a light, externally orientated hypnotic state.

The case could be made that an athlete during an experience of peak performance is actually in a hypnosis-like state. For example, when athletes describe moments of great achievement on the field they often say they feel as if there's a tremendous distortion and time seems to go very slowly. They also often feel as if there were a tunnel vision and they have an immense feeling of relaxation and integration. We saw in the last chapter how David Cone can go into this state when pitching. The upshot is that being in the zone seems to be similar, if not identical, to being in a light, externally oriented hypnotic state.

If athletes become more adept at putting themselves into that kind of hypnotic state, therefore, it will be easier for them to get into the zone and they won't have to keep their fingers crossed or rely on certain rituals prior to their performance in order to do so.

Like peak experiences, what has been called the *flow experience* also shares these qualities with the hypnotic experience. A flow experience is like the peak experience described above, but it extends in time and is more ongoing—ideal for any athlete.

In summary, alert hypnosis is invaluable for athletes in that they don't have to step away from their game, hypnotize themselves for a long period of time in solitude, and then somehow manage to return to the game. That would be entirely impracticable. Using alert hypnosis, athletes can manage their minds by using hypnosis briefly and intermittently throughout a game, or, even better, learn to play while being in a light hypnotic state.

## Eyes open hypnosis

To this end, it is important for the hypnotherapist to know how to create an eyes open hypnotic experience. We teach this to our athletes by first having them do it in an office session. They are then instructed to practice on their own at home. After that, they're instructed to try it during sports practice sessions and then finally to experiment with it during a game.

The protocol for eyes open hypnosis goes like this. First, explain that the induction will be conducted while the athlete has her eyes open. Secondly, be sure to have the athlete focus on something symbolic, away from anything that will make movement. This is because movement creates mental activity and can distract. It is important that the focus of attention be something symbolic because in that way you're making a second intervention. For example, an athlete who needs to develop more strength and power might focus on a picture of a train on the wall. An athlete who needs to spend more time setting and orienting toward goals could focus on some trophy or medal across the room. At this point, ideas for relaxation and other induction suggestions can be given.

The third step is for the therapist to suggest tunnel vision and then use the *development* of tunnel vision for deepening and ratification. You can suggest tunnel vision by mentioning that the person might imagine that she is looking through the cardboard core of a paper-towel roll or through some other such tube. Believe it or not, it's fairly easy to discern when a person is actually evidencing tunnel vision by observing her eyes. Once you notice from her facial expressions and from her eyes that she is having tunnel vision, you can deepen and ratify by mentioning something to the effect that this is evidence that she is responding quite nicely and that she is beginning to go into a wonderful hypnotic state. That ratification allows then for some deepening whereby you can suggest that the athlete use this experience as a vehicle to go even deeper into hypnosis.

Fourth, it's very helpful to suggest that the eyes can defocus a little. As that takes place you can give more suggestions for deepening along these lines: "As your eyes defocus while you remain aware of things around the room in general, you can go even more deeply into hypnosis".

At this point the hypnotherapist can give whatever suggestions are needed about play and performance in general while the subject remains in an eyes open hypnotic state.

Athletes who want to use eyes open hypnosis in competition can aspire to that level of competence and can use what seems to be taking place for some great athlete at the moment. For example, the champion golfer Tiger Woods seems to be extremely focused, as if he had a tunnel vision, when he is entering a golf match. This seems to give him an advantage over other competitors and this can probably be replicated with our ideas. Another great athlete from a different sport, basketball's Michael Jordan, always seemed to be in a different place from his counterparts. It was as if he were able to go beyond the achievements of other athletes and one can speculate that he may have been using techniques of eyes open hypnosis naturally and automatically.

## Talking in hypnosis

After the athlete has had an opportunity to practice eyes open hypnosis on her own, and while playing, it is then time to teach her how to talk in hypnosis—even while playing the game. To teach your subject how to talk in hypnosis, first inform her that people can do this. It's very important to emphasize the "remaining in hypnosis" part of this phrase. In fact it's even helpful to start by saying, "While you remain in hypnosis, you can talk". This is necessary so that the subject does not come out of hypnosis unnecessarily, thinking that's the only way in which she could possibly speak. Some people won't understand if you simply ask them to speak, not knowing that they can do that in hypnosis. So it is essential to reiterate and emphasize the "remain in" part.

A second step can be to suggest that the subject might even find herself going even more deeply into hypnosis as she speaks. There's some tendency, at least at first, for people to go into a lighter state of hypnosis when they speak, because of the need to think more and to be physically active in order to speak. However, as the subjects gain more experience with this technique (and for highly suggestible subjects, right from the start) they can learn to go more deeply into hypnosis as they perform the vocal dialogues.

Having suggested that the subject can not only talk while remaining in hypnosis but can also go even more deeply into hypnosis as she speaks, the therapist can then say, "Tell me what you're experiencing now." It is important to use the term "experiencing" because if you ask people what they are feeling they will talk about their affects, and if you ask them what they are thinking you'll get too many cognitions. So, accordingly, we emphasize the word "experiencing" so that the subject can report in an unbiased way whatever she perceives in her awareness.

Sometimes, even frequently, subjects new to this procedure have difficulty beginning to speak, or give a minimal response. Inasmuch as the experience of physical inertia and the experience of minimal responses is highly typical of the hypnotic state, the hypnotherapist should use any observation of these responses as an opportunity to ratify the development and deepening of the state. Observing these events taking place provides an opportunity to let the client know that she is responding and is moving in the correct direction. Ratification, of course, allows an opportunity to educate as well as to let the client know she is responding properly. This gives a social reinforcement to the client for cooperating.

From this modest beginning of talking about simply what she is experiencing, the client can begin to answer many other questions. This can then lead to her experimenting with eyes open and talking hypnosis in her day-to-day life, and then eventually to the practice field and the game field.

Mrs. Elizabeth Erickson (Milton's wife) was an excellent hypnotic subject and actually preferred to go into hypnosis with her eyes open. She would stare at her diamond engagement ring, slowly defocus her eyes and go into a very deep hypnotic state. While she was in that state, Dr. Erickson and others could ask her about her hypnotic experience and she would describe it. Hypnotically she would have to counteract the tendency to speak more slowly and laboriously, which is exactly the kind of adjustment that people learn to make so that they can appear "normal" to others while being hypnotized. Mrs. Erickson used this technique in hypnotizing herself in the presence of others but it was for her, as it is for others, a perfect way to do self-hypnosis.

Talking in hypnosis is a valuable skill for the athletes to learn for a number of reasons. First of all, to maintain the hypnotic, "in-the-zone" mindset throughout a game, the athlete will need to do so while speaking. Hence it is invaluable to not have to exit the hypnotic state to speak. Athletes, of course, need to speak a lot during most of their performances. Also, team leaders often need to speak to the players, whether it's the basketball guard calling a play or the quarterback calling an audible. Talking is a necessary part of playing. Because hypnosis allows for better performance on the field, hypnosis combined with the ability to talk is invaluable. Also, in the hypnotic state, people are commonly much more creative, so for athletes to be able to strategize and to call plays while remaining hypnotized, they'll be better able to be creative in figuring out ways to deal with the opposition. Furthermore, in many sports, talking trash is designed to fluster and rattle an opponent. If an athlete learns how to talk in hypnosis, he or she will be able to banter while remaining unflappable.

In many ways, eyes open talking hypnosis is a critical part of being "in the zone". When the athlete is in the zone it's as if she were able to perform without any thinking or planning. She responds naturally and very competently to whatever situation arises.

# *Walking in hypnosis*

The third element in alert hypnosis is to train the subject to move while being hypnotized. This can start with walking and progress, of course, to running, jumping, climbing, or whatever. The first step is to inform the person that he can move and walk while remaining hypnotized. Then you should suggest to him that he get up and walk to a symbolic place and then return to the chair in the therapy office. This is a small trial that allows the athlete to sample in an easy-to-do way the experience of moving while hypnotized.

Sometimes people have difficulty beginning to move, or when they start to move they do so slowly and in a cataleptic fashion. The hypnotist at that point should explain any initial difficulties as being indicative of a very highly hypnotized subject inasmuch as this is a sign of the classic hypnotic marker of inertia. Likewise, the hypnotist should also explain the existence and depth of the hypnotic trance by noting that slow or cogwheel-like movements are indicative of this kind of a full response. Explaining this allows the subject not to be disconcerted by hypnotic events that may seem strange compared with events in everyday life. Moreover, it allows him to appreciate the fact that, far from being a distraction, it's wholly indicative of something good.

It's often useful at this point for the hypnotist to use talking in trance to help the subject process and discuss his experiences while walking in trance. If he takes a while to start speaking or speaks slowly or uses only a couple of words, you can of course, explain that as well. Talking in trance affords both subject and operator an opportunity to develop walking in trance as a hypnotic experience and then also to fine-tune it as needed. The fine tuning might involve having the person react more quickly to requests for movement or learn to move more quickly once he's under way, or it might involve his learning how to undo some of the tunnel vision that is very commonly found in eyes open and walking hypnosis. These modifications to what typically arises during hypnotic experiences of having eyes open, walking, and talking are often needed for an athlete to learn how to play his sport while being hypnotized. These modifications are easily made once the subject becomes familiar with the hypnotic experiences in question. First he needs to get started; then in collaboration with you, modifications can be made.

The final step is for the hypnotist to prescribe that the athlete practice this walking in hypnosis at home. First the subject should practice putting himself into a light hypnotic state and walking across the room, and then eventually proceed to doing many of his household tasks and chores in hypnosis. Later, he can not only do that but also relate to other family members and friends while being in hypnosis. The more he expands his abilities to function in hypnosis, the easier it will be for him to call upon this as a resource in practice, and then in games, such that they can easily and effortlessly and fluidly slip into "the zone".

There are many times when being able to walk or perform while in the hypnotic state would be useful. One example would be with an equestrian who is jumping fences and has a long approach to the final one. This was the case in the 2000 Olympics in the showjumping competition. Sometimes, course designers create a very long approach to the final fence to test the mettle of horse and rider. The long approach requires incredible poise because there is the temptation to make too many adjustments to get it right. Having a long time to think can often be the nemesis of the athlete. Athletes, and in this case equestrians, who go into a hypnotic state will be able to access whatever psychological resources are needed in order to perform at their best.

Subjectively, the hypnotic state is characterized by a feeling of inner peace, which creates a performance state best described as embodying poise. Other psychological resources can be easily called up in the hypnotic state. Patience, the hypnotic phenomena of time distortion (psychologically shortening the time to that final fence), and other needed qualities can be accessed and brought forth. So, whether it's the long approach to the final fence when a rider needs to "sit chilly", or not trying too hard or being too casual when you have a breakaway lay-up, there are many times when being in a hypnotic state is useful.

When an equestrian or any other athlete is in the zone it is as if he had naturally accessed the hypnotic state and found that he is automatically able to perform the way he would prefer. I (TR) can remember being in the zone in a high school basketball game. It was as if all I had to do was jump and I knew the shot was going to go in. I felt as if no one could stop me and all I needed was an opportunity to be passed the ball in the right place. When in this state, it's as if the crowd didn't exist, the opposition were not a factor, and the only reality were the execution of the play, shot, or whatever is taking place at the moment. When in the zone, no one wants the experience to end.

The trick for the athlete is how to do this purposefully when it is not accessed spontaneously. This is where the sport psychologist can work with the athlete during a hypnotic session and help him instill an associational cue that can be used "automatically" to re-access being in the zone or the hypnosis-like state. This cue could be a word, a touch, a sound, or any phenomenon that would help bring back the hypnosis-like state on call.

A good example of cues to go automatically into a hypnotic state during a performance occurs in Erickson's work with biathletes. Biathletes are those who ski and then shoot rifles at targets. They get ten shots and are rated in part on their accuracy. Athletes often have difficulty after making seven out of seven, or eight out of eight, because they get nervous, knowing that, with two more bull's-eyes, they would fair well. So it's very common for these athletes to make the first shots and then have a few misses. Of course, in practice, when there is no medal on the line, it is common for them to make ten out of ten. Erickson, in working with biathletes hypnotically, suggested to them that each shot could trigger an amnesia for all prior shots. Then the ninth shot, in the athletes mind, was as if it were the first. This removed all pressure from the athlete. Erickson suggested that it would be only after the tenth shot that the athlete would know to move on to the next set of targets and would ski away accordingly. This is a very good example of a built-in associational cue to go into hypnosis and to utilize the hypnotic phenomena of amnesia. Erickson accomplished it by giving it as a posthypnotic suggestion during his one-on-one work in the office with the athlete. It is often very helpful for the sports psychologist to give a posthypnotic suggestion that something that will *inevitably* occur during the competition or event will *automatically* trigger the hypnotic state and other associated interventions as well.

The work of Milton Erickson is replete with instances of his using eyes open, talking, and walking hypnosis to help his patients. Some of these patients were athletes. We teach it to you just as Erickson taught it to the therapists studying hypnosis with him. He had a very interesting way of teaching it to his students. He would sometimes take a student in one of the classes and meet with her prior to the seminar. He would get her to agree to be a part of an experiment. He would then hypnotize her and suggest she open her eyes, talk, and walk as if she were in the normal waking state while remaining deeply hypnotized all the while. When they arrived for his workshop, Erickson would be quick to challenge the entire class to figure out which student was the hypnotized one. In his initial experiments with this, students could sometimes figure out who was hypnotized because she spoke or moved a little more slowly than the other attendees. That led Erickson to emphasize to the volunteer prior to the seminar that she should move and speak as quickly as a person in the everyday state. He would emphasize that it might not feel natural at first while being in the hypnotized state, but she should make a concerted effort.

No matter how you develop your mastery of eyes open, talking, and walking hypnosis, you can learn to teach it to your clients.

Here is a summary of suggestions that should make your mastery of this material easier.

# *Summary of alert hypnosis*

## *Eyes open hypnosis*

1.  Explain that the induction will be an eyes open one.

2.  Have the client focus on something symbolic, away from anything that will make movement and distract him. Begin suggestions for relaxation.

3.  Suggest tunnel vision and use its development for deepening and ratification.

4.  And/or suggest a defocusing of the eyes—then suggestions for deepening.

## *Talking in hypnosis*

1.  Inform your subject that people *can* talk while remaining in hypnosis.

2.  Then suggest to the subject that she can remain hypnotized or go even more deeply into hypnosis as she speaks.

3.  "Tell me what you are experiencing now."

4.  Explain any difficulty in beginning to speak or any sluggish responses.

## *Walking in hypnosis*

1.  Inform subject that people *can* move and walk while remaining hypnotized.

2. Suggest to him that he can get up and walk to a symbolic place (you specify) and then come back.

3. Explain any difficulty he may experience in moving.

4. Use talking while he's hypnotized to discuss experiences and explain them.

5. Have them practice at home.

# Chapter Seven
# *Hypnotic Phenomena for Intervention in Sport Psychology*

Hypnotic phenomena are cognitive talents that, while evident in everyday life, can most easily be accessed and developed using hypnosis. They have a myriad applications for the athlete. Now we will describe each of the hypnotic phenomena and give some sample applications to illustrate the range of possibilities in sports.

## *Memory functions*

### *Amnesia*

There are three different memory functions that can be used and elicited as hypnotic phenomena to help the athlete change. These are amnesia, hypermnesia and posthypnotic suggestions.

Sport contains a multitude of opportunities to utilize amnesia to help the athlete to perform better. One example would be the athlete who has a horrible game and then, of course, must go and play more games. So many athletes are haunted by a bad game and it continues to stick in their craw in such a way that one bad game becomes a multitude of bad games. Having a negative expectation can really sink a player. We are reminded here of Debbie Thomas's coach, who, prior to her figure-skating perform-ance in the Olympics, cautioned her on her need to do better than her adversary, Katarina Witt. He said, "One mistake, Debbie, and it's all over." Debbie, of course, went onto the ice and made many, many more mistakes than just one! Setting up a negative expectation or carrying one with you in your mind invariably sets the stage for more problems.

So, for the athlete who has had a bad game and doesn't want to be haunted by it, if you elicit amnesia in hypnosis and then point it straight at that terrible event, the athlete will be able to move forward unencumbered.

It's important, whenever you elicit amnesia, first of all to have the person learn any important lesson that needs to be derived from the problematic experience, so that it can be precluded in the future and the person can become a better athlete because of it. Once the lesson has been learned and is remembered subconsciously, the person can afford to forget the catastrophe.

Another example of when we have used amnesia for intervention in sports psychology was when one of our associates came to us for supervision so he could help a school for which he was a consultant to shoot better foul shots. The school had an ongoing history of doing very poorly at the foul line. In his group induction, he emphasized the notion of a fresh start, suggesting that the start of every game could allow the team to forget about all prior games and especially anything having to do with foul shooting. In sports, it is sometimes quite convenient to have a "short memory" on demand.

An interesting example of the use of amnesia in a type of self-hypnosis—or at least a type of self-suggestion—occurred when an American football free safety was being interviewed on a major sports channel. Now bear in mind that free safeties need an unending amount of bravado in order to continue to play at their best. So they can ill afford to remember having been beaten on a pass play because it would deflate them and compromise their performance in the future. This particular free safety kept insisting that he had never ever been beaten. The interviewer knew that he was only half serious but played with him by showing some film of times when a receiver had beaten him long. The free safety merely smiled and said incredulously that someone had stolen his uniform and was impersonating him and insisted again that he had never been beaten!

I (JHE) worked with a golfer once who would feel a tremendous amount of pressure as the game went on, regardless of whether he was doing well or poorly. If he was doing well, he would begin to think about how well he could do and how he could win. If he was doing poorly, he would put too much pressure on himself to get back into the game. It was a case of "damned if you do, damned if you don't" for him psychologically and he was rarely at peace. I used amnesia in hypnosis with this athlete so that, every time that he placed the ball on the tee to tee off, he would instantaneously develop an amnesia for all prior holes. His score-card, while on his person, was forgotten for the time being. This example also illustrates how amnesia can be combined with posthypnotic suggestion to kick in at just the right time.

We saw in Chapter Six how Milton Erickson once used amnesia with biathletes so that they could allow each and every shot to trigger an amnesia for every prior shot. He therefore eloquently removed any pressure from them because every shot was the "first" shot and they could always make one out of one without feeling any kind of pressure to go for ten out of ten.

## Hypermnesia

Hypermnesia is the hypnotic phenomenon that creates perfect re-call—the so-called photographic memory. Hypermnesia is an invaluable resource for athletes who either generate it easily or can be taught to generate it. One example of the use of hypermnesia in sport psychology occurs when athletes are helped to remember vividly the moments of a peak performance. These peak performances serve as reference experiences that the athlete can go back to again and again. Being a recreational equestrian, I (JHE) made a point of flash-freezing moments of near-perfect performance in my mind from all of the years in which I have trained. So they form a collage of sorts that, taken as a whole, gives me a very real and vivid reference point for what I want to attain on a given day. So much of riding involves a "feel" and a combination of different factors. To have these in a composite form in one's mind enables one intuitively, and from a very deep and heartfelt level, to intend a certain result and allow the mind and body to rally that cause.

Another example of the use of hypermnesia concerns learning brand new skills as an athlete. I (JHE) recently began using a personal trainer to learn the proper methods of weightlifting and strength conditioning. Some of the exercises were brand-new and some were old, but, were being taught in a different way from that which I had learned. Frankly, I had learned some really bad weightlifting habits as a football player in high school. So, with some exercises, I not only needed to learn the proper way of lifting but to also *un*learn an old and counterproductive way of lifting. To hold onto the teaching from one weekly session to another, I would purposely put myself in a light self-hypnotic state. Then, while I was being instructed, I would allow the words of the instructor to combine with the feel of the barbells and dumbbells to make an indelible and permanent imprint on my mind. I gave that suggestion and instruction to myself and subsequently had a psychological book of exercises that contained images and feelings and tactile kinesthetic experiences. That psychological book complemented the written material that the personal trainer was generating for me.

## Posthypnotic suggestion

Posthypnotic suggestion involves suggesting to your athlete/ client (or, in the case of self-hypnosis, to yourself) that a certain emotional, psychological, or physical experience will kick in given a certain cue. The cue should be objective and inevitable so that the experience being posthypnotically suggested definitely does occur. In other words, it makes no sense to suggest to a golfer that, when he cleans his ball, an experience of poise will come over him if he cleans his balls infrequently or his caddie does it for him. That's a hit-or-miss approach to something that needs to be more predictable. Instead, it would make more sense to suggest that when he first touches his club, he will get a feeling of settledness and poise. Since he's not going to be hitting anything without a club, we know that is an inevitable cue that we can count on. It's important to remember also that the more vivid and sensory the posthypnotic cue is, the more effective it is likely to be. For example, if a baseball player is told he can have a certain experience upon smelling the leather of his glove, or a hitter is told that he can remember and experience his foot moving forward in the batter's box (the antithesis of "bailing out" when hitting) upon feeling the pine tar on his hands, then that will be more likely to be effective than a suggestion that is contingent upon something less compelling.

One example of giving oneself posthypnotic suggestions occurred when I (JHE) was nervous about going into one of my first horse shows. I suggested to myself that upon entering the ring I would ride and feel as if I were the world-famous equestrian, Mark Leone. (Parenthetically, I can say I purposely chose a larger rider such as myself so that the identification would be somewhat more realistic.) The intervention worked wonderfully when I entered the ring but I had totally forgotten to consider the fact that I would be warming up for half an hour prior to ever getting there! My warm-up—or schooling session, as it is called—was a disaster! I was sure for the next show to suggest to myself that when I entered the show ground I would take on the persona of Mark Leone. Having done that, both the schooling session and the competitive rounds in the ring worked out well.

# Hypnotic phenomena and time

## Time contraction

Time contraction is the hypnotic phenomenon that allows a long period to be experienced psychologically as very brief. This can often be useful for athletes. One example would be a jockey waiting in the gate a long time for the horses to be loaded. This often proves problematic, because what the spectator might think is just a couple of minutes seems like a long time to the jockey, and he can often lose his focus and edge, as can the horse. He needs to keep his edge and then keep his horse alert. With time contraction suggested either in an office session or in a self-hypnotic moment by the jockey himself, that long period of time can seem like only seconds. In that way, the mental sharpness can be maintained. Often, the larger the race, the more important this becomes. The Kentucky Derby, with huge fields of up to twenty, often necessitates something of this order so the horses and jockeys who have been loaded early will be ready to run when the gates open.

Time contraction also becomes valuable to someone like a field goal kicker who is preparing to kick an important field goal only to find that the opposing team has called a timeout to "ice" him. The passing minutes during the timeout, can seem interminable to a field goal kicker.

The same phenomenon occurs in soccer prior to a penalty shot and would also occur when a timeout has happened before an important free throw in basketball. When an athlete suggests to herself that time can pass as if the hands of the clock were whipping around its face and that everything is moving quite rapidly, then that will afford her the opportunity to experience the subjective phenomenon of time in a way that is most useful to her as an athlete.

In equestrian pursuits, some people go around a jumper course too slowly. They can be liable for what are called "time faults", which means that the outer limit that is allowed for the round is exceeded and they are penalized. For riders who chronically experience this kind of problem, time contraction can be very useful in that it can give them the subjective sense that time is passing more quickly and can get them to hustle things along a little bit more. It would allow them to balance out their natural tendency to experience time as being elongated by collapsing time down and thereby developing an acute awareness of just how fast it is moving. This would help them to complete their round within the allowed time.

## Time expansion

Time expansion or elongation involves the subjective experience of clock time as taking much longer than it does. In everyday life, people experience time elongation when they are doing things such as waiting for water to boil or for a late train to come. In situations like that, a couple of minutes seems like half an hour. How can this be used to help athletes? Well, suppose a basketball player has a tendency to rush his shot when there are only a few seconds left on the clock. Elite athletes know that even a few seconds of clock time can be used to the fullest and that they don't need to rush or force a shot precipitately. They learn just how to use every split second. But other athletes aren't so gifted and they can use hypnotic phenomena—in particular the hypnotic phenomenon of time elongation—to give themselves a subjective sense that they have more time than they thought they did. The basketball player who rushes a shot can be taught to experience things as if he were in a time warp and time were moving at half the normal speed. This can be suggested to him in a sport psychology session proper or taught as a self-hypnosis skill to be used as needed.

Equestrians who ride the jumpers have sixty seconds upon entering the ring to start their round. Nervous or novice riders do not use that full amount of time to their advantage. What they should be doing is taking their time walking around, relaxing their horse, relaxing themselves, and very importantly, giving their horses sneak peeks at some of the more daunting fences. A rider who starts her round prematurely robs herself and her horse of all these advantages, to their detriment. If riders who habitually make that mistake are taught to elongate time, they will take more of it, knowing that they have so much more than they thought. Altering the perception of time hypnotically allows the athlete to counteract some of her natural and hindering tendencies such that she can perform to her potential.

## Age regression

Age regression occurs when the athlete is taken back in time to re-experience various athletic endeavors so that they can be re-vivified and re-experienced. Hypnotic age regression is ideal for helping athletes to retrieve any past psychological resource that would facilitate their present performance. For example, an athlete who has been soundly defeated in a contest may be full of doubt and despair. She can be taken back in time to when she manifested immense resiliency. This would enable her to bounce back more quickly than would be the case if she hadn't had the hypnotic intervention. Another example would be that of an athlete who is having a string of bad luck and it looks as if his career isn't going to progress as he hoped. He can be taken back in time to a point when he showed great determination on the ball field.

Know that it's helpful to take athletes back to numerous times when these resources were in evidence. And also know that it's actually very important that you take them back in time to moments when the resources were being manifested in their rudimentary form, not necessarily when they first appeared in a full-blown way. For example, to aid determination, it could be helpful to take a baseball player back to when he was playing stickball and the pitcher was an older boy on the street and was about to strike him out for the third straight time. The focus of the eye, the lock of the jaw, the tenacity in the body language—all these things remembered again will allow an older ballplayer to stick with it.

Another example of age regression in action could be the cultivation of the ability to be calm under pressure or to have poise. A hypnotherapist can identify one, two, or three different experiences where poise was present. Better yet, the hypnotherapist can request of an independently thinking patient in hypnosis that he take himself back to times in his personal life and in his athletic life when he experienced this sense of presence. It doesn't even need to be solely times when athletics were being played. For example, someone could go back in time to when he was playing "pick-up-sticks" as a child. Just about everyone can remember cultivating on-the-spot poise as they went to reach for a stick that was precariously perched and yet could be pulled out with patience and a steady hand.

Athletes can often benefit from cultivating a positive expectation of their upcoming performance. Milton Erickson had an intervention that he called the *early-learning set induction*, which involved helping a person to remember all of the details of when she first learned the alphabet. In starting the induction, he highlighted the doubt that we all had in learning our ABCs. In emphasizing the doubt and then, on the heals of that, emphasizing how we did, in fact, learn how to make letters and then numbers, and then learned how to write in cursive script, he reminded his patients that they could succeed in spite of any doubts, and that their sub-conscious mind had capabilities that their conscious mind wasn't always aware of. Doing this for athletes would afford them the opportunity to override doubts the conscious mind has and help them to recognize that their bodies know a lot more than their minds do, and can succeed accordingly.

A perfect example of using age regression to develop a positive expectation occurred when Christian Laettner was in the NCAA basketball tournament and his team, the heavily favored Duke Blue Devils, were down by one point with just a couple of seconds left in the game. Laettner received the ball at the top of the key, and was very fortunate to have a long inbound pass reach him without incident. He still had an incredibly long shot to make but, with his sense of poise and sense of positive expecta-tion, he faked in one direction and then whirled in the other direction delivering a buzzer-beating jump shot. Later he was asked in the locker room how he developed such a sense of confi-dence and also whether he was nervous. He said he wasn't nerv-ous and had developed his sense of confidence by mentally reviewing all the times in grade school and high school where he had received the ball in a clutch situation and had made this very same or a similar kind of shot. Christian Laettner put himself into a type of self-hypnotic reverie and did a very rapid age regression to numerous examples of what he was about to do. This also illus-trates the misconception that sport psychology and hypnosis takes a long time to be effective. In this example, it was done within a matter of moments and right on the spot as needed.

## Age progression

Age progression is the complement of age regression. By now you may have noticed that some of the hypnotic phenomena tend to come in pairings. For example, amnesia has as its complement hypermnesia. Time contraction has as its complement time elon-gation or expansion. Age progression is a subjective experience to the person moving forward in time to experience elements of a wished-for future. Unlike age regression, progression obviously does not entail going to experiences that are "objectively real" as age regression does. Age progression moves forward in time to help athletes to experience what they would like to achieve. For example, in my (TR's) work with high school soccer athletes, I suggest that, while in an altered state of consciousness, players project themselves into the day after the game. This takes place as part of a process that involves their psychological preparation for an upcoming contest. They are then asked to imagine reading about their victory in their local newspaper. From that vantage point, they are asked to review what they and their team-mates did that contributed to their win. They are then asked to memorize these recorded events and bring them back to the present and link them to their current game plan for mastery and success.

# *Dissociation*

Dissociation is the psychological capability of a person to separate herself from an experience or from a feeling. Most of the time, as therapists, we encounter dissociation when it's being used by a person counterproductively in her life, as is the case with dissociative disorders. But dissociation is a neutral psychological capability that can be used for something either positive or negative. An example of a positive use of dissociation is when the surgeon cuts open the patient, and despite all sorts of blood and gore, is able to operate with composure. This individual has been able to separate his feelings from his cognitive capabilities so as to remain utterly cool, unlike those of us who haven't been trained as surgeons. Without dissociation, this person would, like the rest of us, cringe at the sight!

We have used dissociation with our athletes in a number of different ways. One example would be with the athlete who is having personal problems. Whether they are financial or familial troubles, athletes need to put aside these everyday woes in order to perform on the field. When athletes are haunted by what is going on in their personal lives, it invariably compromises their game. But, of course, this is true for the game of life as well as for the athletes we work with. Who among us hasn't had to push off to the side an argument or fight with a spouse or partner when there's something else that needs to be done? As therapists, we can't be working with our patients while we are ruminating about some situation at home. Of course, it's often with our athletes that the need to accomplish these things becomes most evident. Whereas people can squeak by without doing the things we're talking about in this chapter day in and day out, often the athlete is forced to accomplish these things psychologically, or else it would be very compromising.

Another example of using dissociation in sports occurs with the athlete whose injury has been diagnosed and treated and she knows it won't get worse and yet she is favoring it on the field. Perhaps she is not only favoring it but also worrying about the pain she experiences, unnecessarily. Once this type of player has received full medical assurance that she can play through the pain without additional injury, she can choose to dissociate from the pain itself. If she doesn't, her performance will no doubt be compromised, whether it's a matter of "hearing footsteps" out of fear of getting hit in that spot again or favoring it in such a way that her mechanics change. When the player develops the ability to separate herself totally from that part of her body, then her performance will remain uncompromised by what is going on. It is only when pain is a signal that diagnosis and treatment are needed that we must allow for it in our minds.

There are a couple of interesting examples of what can happen to athletes when they are unable to dissociate from some aspect of their life. Mark Wohlers was perhaps the most dominating closer in all of baseball. His fast ball frequently approached 100 miles per hour and batters were utterly intimidated by his presence. Yet shortly after he was divorced, longing for the children who were often away from him, he began to develop some problems with his control. These problems snowballed to the extent that he had to go down to the minor leagues and was injured there. He himself repeatedly pointed to his family problems as being the cause of his athletic difficulties. He represented himself as a very emotionally sensitive man who was very troubled by what was happening with his family to the point where he couldn't perform with a clear mind.

Another example of an athlete who has been haunted by something that he couldn't dissociate from is former Yankee second baseman Chuck Knobluck. Having a history of botching throws from second base to first base, Knobluck has nonetheless gone through long periods of time where his throws have been a nonissue, and yet, once he makes an error of this nature, it seems like it not only rains but pours. Clearly, a new error precipitates an awful lot of thinking about prior errors. If Chuck Knobluck were able to develop the hypnotic ability to dissociate, then he could be left with only his history of good throwing with the effect that he would be focused on what he wants to do instead of worrying about what he is terrified of once again doing.

## *Hypnotic dreaming and daydreaming*

Hypnotic dreaming and daydreaming involves the athlete's ability to have a dream or a daydream that makes a contribution to his positive mindset. This can happen either in the hypnosis proper or at night when he is asleep. Athletes can be encouraged either to dream about a success or to dream about experiencing something that they are developing in their game. For example, a pitcher who is trying to develop a change-up and hasn't yet experienced it might find himself experiencing it for the first time in a dream. Likewise, athletes can solve certain dilemmas that they are faced with in terms of strategy vis-à-vis the other team.

The history of the world is filled with scientists and creative people who have discovered something in their dreams. An example would be Einstein, who, as a boy, dreamed or daydreamed about riding a long stream of light at the *speed* of light and then of course later worked on how this could be. The American biochemist James Watson and the British biophysicist Francis Krick were stumped as to how the genetic code could be structured in physiology. One of them had a dream one night about two snakes twisted around each other and that became the basis of their discovery about the double-stranded helix that describes the shape of the DNA molecule.

Having taken years off from riding as an equestrian, Janet Edgette knew that she had to go back to it when, night after night, she would have vivid dreams of jumping over large fences. The dreams were so vivid that she could feel the horse underneath her and could feel the loft as they soared through the air. It was at once totally exhilarating and even more totally compelling, such that it created an irresistible urge to ride. Dreams afford us the opportunity to listen more closely to what our subconscious mind is telling us.

Hypnotic dreaming can also be employed to solve strategic problems. For example, a team who has a very tough defense to score against might seem a daunting opponent in the week prior to the contest. So long as only the conscious mind is trying to figure out how to score, the person is only using half or less than half of his mental capacity. A hypnotic dream could provide some hints of new plays or new approaches that could help develop a different strategy.

Hypnotic dreaming and daydreaming could provide a useful alternative to age progression in giving the athlete a sense of positive expectation that something is inevitably going to happen. So the athlete plagued by doubt could have a dream about his soon-to-be victory. Whether it is an experience of being carried off on the shoulders of other players, the vivid appearance of the scoreboard with the black background and the tiny lights lit up, or the refreshing feeling of the shower after the victory—whatever the dream, these experiences can instill a tremendous sense of hope and confidence. Who has not had an inspiring dream and then felt the emotional tenor of that dream continue into the day and even the week?

## Dissociated movement

### Catalepsy

Catalepsy is the experience of one's body, usually the arm and hand, as being warm, heavy and often numb in hypnosis.

Fortunately, this state, which is induced through suggestion, can be re-experienced when needed outside of hypnosis. While this may sound strange to readers who don't have much experience of hypnosis and perhaps feel it would be difficult to induce, catalepsy is actually so very easy to bring about that it often occurs naturally as a part of the hypnotic state. That is to say, catalepsy often appears as a by-product of hypnosis even if it hasn't been specifically suggested.

I (JHE) once worked with a chess player in Croatia who complained that when he was in the midst of a match he would become too impulsive and move his piece prematurely. He needed to learn how to wait and think a little bit more and pick up his hand and move his piece when the time was right. My main intervention for him in hypnosis, and in the self-hypnosis that I subsequently taught him, was to show him how to make his hand cataleptic so it would lie on the table more easily and move only when he was certain that the time was right. I gave him the posthypnotic suggestion that, any time he was feeling anxious and impulsive, catalepsy could return to him in a flash and his hand could remain on the table for as long as was needed.

This same hypnotic phenomena of catalepsy could be used with a basketball player who is about to foul out and needs to remind herself to keep her hands away from the opposing player so she doesn't get called for her next foul. Likewise, for a lineman who jumps offside prior to the snap of the ball, catalepsy can help him remain on side even with a short count.

## Ideomotor movement (arm levitation)

Arm levitation happens when your arm becomes light and moves into the air in an effortless way. This phenomenon is often experienced as *avolitional*, that is, the arm is moving autonomously, without volition.

One example of arm levitation in use with a sportsman occurred when I (JHE) worked with a man who had dogs that engaged in trials whereby they were judged on their ability to move around a field based on signals from the trainer's hand. The dog and trainer were so good that they would often get to the national competitions. But, time and time again, anxiety and pressure would translate into a hand tremor in the trainer, so that he was inadvertently making tiny finger signals to the dog that he didn't intend and thereby sending the dog off course, resulting in a loss. In hypnosis, I combined some catalepsy (so that the fingers remained still) with arm levitation (so that it would move into the air), with the end result that the trainer was able to make only the movements that he intended and none of the movements that would have been dictated by the experience of anxiety in his arm. The catalepsy kept the fingers still while the arm levitation allowed the arm to move into the air and also be still.

Ideomotor movement can also be evidenced in automatic finger signaling in hypnosis. This enables the athlete to communicate without having to speak, thereby often making it easier for him to remain in deep hypnosis while communicating with the hypnotherapist. Hypnotists would have no way of knowing whether the subject was complying with a request to go back and re-experience a moment of determination, or a moment of success, if they didn't have some way of communicating with the athlete. Sometimes, by developing a "yes" finger, a "no" finger, and an "I don't know" finger, the athlete can communicate most effectively and the work in hypnosis can be thereby more efficient.

Sometimes arm levitation can be evoked as a veritable symbol of what needs to be done in a literal sense on the field. For example, working with a lineman who is rushing the quarterback, the athlete's complaint was that his coach was always yelling at him to get his hands up to block the passer's view of the field. It was hard for him to remember to do this. In hypnosis, I (JHE) had him develop a dual arm levitation and then suggested to him that any time he was rushing a passer his arms could go up in a similar manner. This enabled him to comply more effectively with his coach's request.

A similar situation occurs in basketball where, on defense, it's very important for the players to keep their hands up so they can block passes more easily and obscure the offensive player's view of the court and the other players. Yet so often it is hard for defensive players to remember this and it's so very common to hear coaches yelling at their defense to put their hands up. To make things a little easier on the coaches and the players, arm levitation could be employed and posthypnotically suggested so that it occurred with greater frequency at all levels of the game.

# Automatic drawing

Automatic drawing is a more complete development of the hypnotic phenomenon that was once referred to as automatic writing. In automatic drawing, the hypnotized athlete is encouraged to draw a picture that would be useful to her as an athlete. She experiences drawing it almost as if it is happening *through* her and not of her own volition. One of our favorite ways of using hypnotic drawing is to have the athlete develop a hypnotic training room. To make a hypnotic training room, the athlete is given a pad and various markers and then is hypnotized. She's told, while remaining in hypnosis, to open her eyes and to draw a rectangle. It is then explained to her that this rectangle is her special training room and she is to draw inside the training room various things that would help her to develop a very good mindset.

Now these items can either be representational or abstract. One athlete might put in her training room a trophy that she won years ago. Another athlete might put in quotations or a coach's inspirational words about his talent. Another person may draw a picture of a scoreboard showing her team having won the big game. Whatever creates in the athlete the winning mental set is to be put inside the training room.

After doing this, the athlete is then instructed to put outside the training room those elements that serve to take her out of her mindset. So on the outside, for a child athlete, it might be the parents complaining about how much their sport costs. For another athlete, outside the training room, might be a picture of a day when she was the "goat". This separation of what is inside from what is outside fosters a dissociation that allows the athlete to keep her focus and not be beleaguered by counterproductive thoughts.

The last element in the athlete's training room is something that separates the inside from the outside and keeps the separation intact. We have had athletes draw pictures of Arnold Schwarzenegger patrolling the boarder as a bouncer such that what's outside stays outside and what is inside stays inside! Other athletes have had Pete Sampras playing doubles and slapping back over the net (training-room wall) anything that is hit in by the opponent. Someone else, a rather small quarterback, had the walls of their training room patrolled by a number of the beefy lineman who would later protect him in the pocket.

The training room and hypnotic drawing in general forms a valuable asset for athletes who are inclined in this direction or could be encouraged to produce these kinds of things. While this may not be for everyone, those who take to it can get a lot of mileage out of it.

## Anesthesia and analgesia

Anesthesia is a loss of sensation, and can, in the case of a general anesthetic, mean a loss of consciousness, too. It can also be local, as when the dental surgeon freezes your gum, or topical, when an anesthetic is, say, sprayed onto the skin to numb just that part of the surface. Analgesia is a reduction in the ability to feel pain, or the relief of pain, often by the use of drugs that block the transmission of nerve impulses. These two phenomena, when induced hypnotically, can, as you can well imagine, prove invaluable when a player needs to play through pain.

It is important, however, that athletes *should not play through hypnotically induced pain relief if by doing so they are exarcebating a problem.* They should consult their physician first. A good example of this situation was when I (JHE) was approached by my aunt, who was a marathon runner. She had terrible knee pain from years of running on hard surfaces. It was so bad, in fact, that she could hardly run on them and was relegated to walking her marathons with the Achilles Heel Roadrunning Club (a group for injured runners). When she came to me (JHE) with the request that I hypnotize her, numb her knees so that she could run in the New York marathon, I asked her what her physician had said about any further running. She said he had told her that, if she continued to run, she would become crippled and unable even to walk. Crazed athlete that she was, she nonetheless wanted to continue to run in the marathons using hypnotic anesthesia. Obviously, I recognized this as an illegitimate use of hypnosis. I spoke to her about the situation and spelled out what she was doing to herself so self-destructively.

Pain is only sometimes a signal that something needs to be diagnosed and treated. Sometimes pain is a healing pain or pain that can, in fact, be played through without damage to the body. In these instances, hypnotic anesthesia or analgesia can be evoked so that the player can continue performing.

I (TR) had a player who sustained a broken toe during a soccer game. He was evaluated by a physician and given clearance to play, even though the toe was broken. Hypnotic anesthesia was used to facilitate pain control. He played the next game and missed only some practice time.

Anesthesia can also be used in a metaphorical or symbolic way. For example, athletes who are too sensitive to a coach's criticism or too short-tempered with the incessant questions that media personnel might ask can be taught to go into a self-hypnotic state and include a numbing of their head as a part of that self-hypnosis. Here, the numbing of the head is a symbolic way of self-suggesting that they be a little bit less sensitive, even *in*sensitive, to some of what is being thrown their way.

I (JHE) can remember moping for months after a big football game that ended in a 0–0 tie after I unfortunately fell on a fumble, thinking that the opposing team were close by and ready to tackle me. At the time, I thought that I just wanted to secure the ball for our offense to take over and try to score. Being a hefty and chunky lineman, I did not think to try to run with the ball and indeed, year after year, we had gotten it drilled into our head simply to fall on the ball and get the posses-sion. But this was in the final seconds and it really was our last hope and—low and behold!—later the videotapes showed that there was hardly a person in sight except for me. Truly, I could have scooped up the ball and run down the field to be the hero of the day against the arch-rival. Unfortunately, I wound up being the goat and I can still remember the coach screaming at me from the sidelines, asking why I didn't pick the ball up and run with it. That moment seemed to last, in a time-distorted way, for the bet-ter part of an hour, and it also seems now and seemed at the time as if the entire stadium of fans could hear every word he said as they glared at me in silence. So, at that time, I certainly could have used this technique of symbolic psychological anesthesia.

It is intriguing to think of all the athletes and coaches who could use this technique of psychological aversion in their relations with the media. Of course, for viewers, it would make for a less interesting newscast! However, fines might be fewer and relationships might be better in the sport. Wouldn't, in fact, the world be a better place if notoriously hot-tempered (and frequently reprimanded) basketball coach, Bobby Knight, learned these techniques? Yet, some would no doubt miss the entertainment value of, for example, watching Jim Everett, the quarterback, attack the interviewer Jim Rome on ESPN after Rome bated him by making a reference to his not being very tough by calling him Chris Evert (the female tennis cham-pion). It might have been quite a stretch of the imagination to have predicted that the baseball player Pete Rose would be able to maintain his composure while being provocatively interviewed by Jim Gray during All-Star festivities in 1999. But he did—uncharacteristically so. Perhaps that's the kind of result that ath-letes and coaches can hope for when employing some of these techniques.

## Hyperesthesia

Hyperesthesia is the hypnotic ability to increase sensation in the body or mind. And, as in the case with anesthesia and analgesia, the changes actually go to the physiological level.

One application of hypnotically induced hyperesthesia could be to a pitcher's or a quarterback's hand after an injury. A loss of sensation could severely impair a pitcher's ability to throw strikes and to use his usual repertoire of pitches, or a quarterback's ability to throw the ball with precision. A similar thing happens in very cold weather: there is a loss of sensation. Another application of hyperesthesia comes in equestrian sports. Here the rider needs to be incredibly sensitive to the horse's movements and the movements of his own body in order to cue the horse. When a rider so much as twitches a muscle in his hand or legs, the horse responds. For example, a light contraction of the calf muscle will send the horse significantly forward, and simply closing one's fingers a quarter of an inch on one of the hands will slow a horse significantly. Some riders are limited in their ability to improve because of insensitivity. For those riders hyperesthesia can be employed to improve their riding.

## *Positive therapeutic hallucinations*

"Positive therapeutic hallucinations" refers to the hypnotic capacity that a person has to see, hear, or touch something that in reality is not there. Here, the word "positive" indicates that, while the thing is not there in reality, you are inserting it. It doesn't refer to the fact that it is a good experience. Since this is the therapeutic employment of hallucinations, it does however invariably result in a good experience.

For example, I (TR) had the good fortunate to play high school basketball for a very talented coach. He was good at understanding both the game and the psychological processes. He once told me that I was a clutch player and that it was my responsibility to take the shot at the end of the game if circumstances warranted. I believed him, trusted him, and, at the time, he was my hero. When the game was on the line, I did as he had told me. I would hear his voice telling me to take the shot, and that I could make this and we would win the game. Incredibly, I cannot remember ever not making a shot that would have meant a difference in a game in college or recreational league play, long after I had ended my playing career with him.

In the movie *The Waterboy* the character played by the actor Adam Sandler imagines that he would hear the voices of those in the past making fun of him. He would then use this as a resource to attack the opposition because he would see and hear these people from the past agitating him. This made him a ferocious football player in the game and he was a hero for the school that he was competing for at that time. Of course, this is the use of visual and auditory hallucination.

Still yet another application of positive hallucinations is with a team that has a very poor record when playing on the road. I (JHE) have helped athletes to hallucinate their home arena or stadium so that they could feel the kind of confidence they experience when playing at home—and play accordingly.

Positive therapeutic hallucinations also can come in handy to change a player's or a team's attitude about the opposition. For example, I (JHE) worked with an offensive lineman who was totally intimidated by a player on one of the other teams who weighed much more than he did and was much stronger. The fact that he was intimidated made the mismatch that much worse. To eliminate his intimidation, I suggested to him in hypnosis that, whenever he saw the player on the field, he would see him wearing diapers, similar to the cartoon character Baby Hughie! Like so many subjects in hypnosis, especially subjects who have mild to moderate hypnotic ability, he half saw it and half didn't see it, but at game time it brought a smile to his face, helped him to relax, and certainly helped him to be less intimidated. This technique actually has its roots in the old coach's adage, "They put their pants on the same way that you do." Or the variation that my high school football coach used: "They look the same sitting on the pot as you do in the morning."

## Negative therapeutic hallucinations

Negative therapeutic hallucinations involve the hypnotized subject's ability to eliminate or remove something that can be seen, heard, or felt in the environment. It is the complement of positive hallucinations. As with positive hallucinations, the adjective should not be taken literally, but in this case refers to the fact that something that is present in reality is being eliminated perceptually. One example of the use of negative hallucinations with athletes occurs when someone consults us who is distracted on the playing field or court. For example, many a foul shooter can lose his poise when the crowd behind the hoop are waving their arms or other distracting objects such as the infamous "terrible towels" that the New York Knicks fans have. Others might be distracted by the annoying placards encouraging television viewers to read passages from the Bible. Therapists employing negative hallucination can suggest in hypnosis, or can have the athlete suggest in self-hypnosis, that the background is blurry, fuzzy, or even all white.

Another application of negative hallucination occurred when I (JHE) worked with a field goal kicker who would get rattled when about to kick an important field goal and the opposition called a timeout. This gave him all too much time to think and listen to the jeering of the crowd. In mentioning this case earlier, I spoke about the time distortion that I had the player do. But I also buttressed that with negative hallucination and suggested to him that not only could he white out the crowd as if there were a terrible snowstorm on one portion of the field, but also that he could hear only silence, as if he had a very bad head cold and his ears were stopped up.

A variation of negative therapeutic hallucination is the induction of tunnel vision in hypnosis. With tunnel vision, the periphery is removed and what is left is what the athlete wants to be attentive to. The induction of negative hallucination in the form of tunnel vision is ideally suited to helping athletes who need to focus better. Many elite athletes do this naturally without the use of hypnosis. However, this is splitting hairs because many elite athletes, of course, slip into "the zone", which is like a natural everyday trance state. An example of this kind of athlete would be David Cone. I (JHE) remember watching Cone during the height of his career, pitching in the World Series. The camera that looked out at the pitcher's mound from behind the catcher captured his face, and his eyes were similar to what a hypnotic subject's eyes would look like when open. The focus and concentration was such that nothing other than the catcher's mitt and the batter were being seen. This same stare could be seen clearly on the face of Mark McGuire during his record-breaking home-run-hitting season. Once he locked in on the pitcher, you could see an intensity of the stare that simply would not allow for anything outside of the pitcher and the ball to be present in his visual sphere.

At this point, it's important that we elucidate a specific protocol through which hypnotic phenomena can be elicited. The protocol is as follows:

1. Seeding

2. Language-based suggestions for the phenomena

    a. Presuppositions
    b. Direct suggestion
    c. Double binds
    d. Conscious/subconscious dissociated statements

3. Metaphors

4. Natural examples from everyday life

5. Symbols

6. Follow-through

# 1. Seeding

The first thing a sport psychologist using hypnosis to elicit hypnotic phenomena can do is *seed* the hypnotic phenomena. Seeding is the hypnotic equivalent of the literary device of foreshadowing. In seeding, you hint at what is to come in the hypnosis proper. Seed prior to the actual hypnotic session and the hypnotic intervention as a way of "priming the pump".

Examples of this method are as follows:

i.   Become very curious about what kind of delight-fully disarming experience you'll have in trance today. (Arm levitation)

ii. As you settle into a comfortable trance depth, your unconscious mind can begin to draw its own conclusions about the
matter at hand. (Automatic drawing)
iii. Wasn't it easy for you to have lost awareness of the traffic
sounds outside? Go ahead and override the needs of your
conscious mind to realize everything and let your unconscious teach you about the beauty and simplicity of absence.
(Negative hallucination)

# 2. *Language-based suggestions*

In the hypnotic work proper, there are four major language-based
ways of eliciting hypnotic phenomena. First, the therapist can use
*presuppositions*. Presuppositions constitute therapeutic assuming.
Here you assume that something is going to happen and therefore
the subject believes accordingly. It is an indirect way of getting the
client to believe that something is true. In so expecting, they will
experience.

Examples of this method are as follows:

i. Your first inkling that a dream is about to take place can
be your cue to go ever more deeply into trance. (Hypnotic
dreaming)
ii. Once you recognize your perception of time/space/sensation
beginning to alter, your unconscious can begin to speculate
about how best to apply that different and special experience of the world. (Time distortion/dissociation/positive
and negative hallucination)
iii. When you first wonder whether it's warmth or numbness you
feel in your hands, you can smile with pride at how well your
body responds to hypnosis. (Catalepsy)

A second language-based way of noticing hypnotic phenomena
is *direct suggestion*. This is the easiest and most obvious method
of eliciting hypnotic phenomena in that you simply and forth-
rightly suggest it. For example, you can suggest that a basketball

player's arms would feel heavy any time he wanted to resist temptation to reach up and unnecessarily foul an opponent he is angry at.

Examples of this method are as follows:

i.   Invite that whimsical part of you to lift your hand – let it enchant you! (Arm levitation)
ii.  Slowly, ever so slowly, slow down inside, and let time follow. (Time distortion)
iii. You, too, can be this imaginary professional athlete, right here, as a grown-up, whether or not you had an imaginary friend or two or three as a child. Why not ask your unconscious mind to open up those memory stores and show you again how easy it is to drum up whomever you need. (Positive visual/auditory hallucination)

*Double binds* constitute the third language-based way in which hypnotic phenomena can be elicited. With double binds you offer an illusion of alternatives. After you have offered such, the client feels a freedom to choose but you've presented two possibilities, either of which moves the client in the desired direction.

Examples of this method are as follows:

i.   Perhaps it will be your left hand that begins to feel light and rise up or maybe it will be your right hand that will feel an increased sense of levity.
ii.  You can develop a deep and profound and robust amnesia for any bad putt that rattles you immediately after you make that putt, or you can develop that immense and unbreachable amnesia the minute you go to make your next putt.
iii. Yes those New York fans are a hostile bunch. And, yes, you have been shaken up in the past by them when playing in Madison Square Garden. But, now that you're receiving hypnosis, this next time will be different. You may either experience an arena filled with empty seats, as if you were practicing long before anyone has arrived, or perhaps see the crowd as being made up of various circus animals all performing: one man might be a seal with a ball on his nose; a woman might be

an elephant balancing on her hind two legs; another young man might be like a parrot relentlessly chanting only what he has been taught, in a repetitive and monotonous and even humorous kind of way.

*Conscious/subconscious dissociative statements* are the fourth and final language-based way in which hypnotic phenomena can be elicited. With these suggestions the client's conscious mind is coaxed to do one productive thing related to a hypnotic phenomenon while her subconscious mind is simultaneously coaxed into doing something complementary, yet different.

Examples of this method are as follows:

i.   Your conscious mind can let go of certain fragments of thoughts while your unconscious mind lets go of entire texts of ideas. (Amnesia)
ii.  Your conscious mind can become aware of feeling wistful while your unconscious mind tenderly reveals an old thought or two that has some bearing on the things we spoke about today. (Hypermnesia)
iii. Your conscious mind can imagine what it feels like to comfortably experience accuracy at the foul line while your unconscious mind thinks about the kinds of conversations you can have with your coach that will lead to that experience. (Future progression)

# 3. *Metaphors*

Metaphors are often very helpful in eliciting hypnotic phenomena. A metaphor in our context is a story or anecdote that contains within it suggestions for the development of the hypnotic phenomenon in question.

Examples of sample metaphors designed to induce a specific hypnotic phenomena are as follows:

i.   Fog lifting, reassembly of jigsaw puzzles, series of knots being untied one by one. (Hypermnesia)

ii.  Circuit breaker, dials, "thick skin". (Anesthesia/analgesia)
iii. Clocks with worn-out batteries, cuckoo clocks with worn-out mechanisms, daylight savings, running through water. (Time expansion)

# 4. *Natural examples*

Natural examples of a hypnosis-like or pseudo-hypnotic nature drawn from everyday life constitute still yet another wonderful way of eliciting hypnotic phenomena. They illustrate the hypnosis that occurs in ordinary life and as such they can show people that the hypnotic phenomena we're seeking to create are not so very unusual but are in fact sometimes part and parcel of our day. While using natural examples, subjects get the sense that they are not producing something alien but instead something familiar.

Examples of natural hypnosis-like situations that can elicit hypnotic phenomena are as follows:

i.   Szechwan chicken, hot salsa, new shoes, professional perfume developers. (Hyperesthesia)
ii.  Physiological habituation to sound/temperature, absorption in a movie to the exclusion of hearing the telephone ring. (Negative hallucination)
iii. Red light/green light childhood game, Simon Says, sprinters at the block, divers poised at the 10-meter board. (Catalepsy)

# 5. *Symbols*

Therapists can use symbols to elicit hypnotic phenomena. When you use a symbol you are using a living representation of the hypnotic phenomenon in question.

Examples of symbols that can be developed in hypnosis to elicit a hypnotic phenomena are as follows:

i.   Mannequin (Arm levitation)
ii.  Elephant toy (Hypermnesia)
iii. Etch-A-Sketch (Automatic drawing)
iv.  Polygraph (Automatic writing)
v.   Nursery rhyme (Age regression)


# 6. *Follow-through*

After making these suggestions designed to produce hypnotic phenomena, it's useful to follow through. Just as following through is an important part of any athletic act, it is important in hypnotic work. Therefore, after the hypnosis proper is over, it is useful to make mention of things that will help to consolidate the intervention that was promoted during the session.

Examples of this method are as follows:

i.   Repeat what was said during the hypnosis.
ii.  Say it in a different way.
iii. Give posthypnotic suggestions to enable the effect to be re-experienced later.
iv.  Make verbal and visual bridges between what occurred in hypnosis and everyday life.
v.   Ask the athlete how she thinks she might use the intervention just suggested in the hypnotic session.

# Chapter Eight
# Changing the "Viewing" and the "Doing" for Athletic Success

By changing the *viewing* of the athletes' situation at hand and/or changing the *doing* of it, both coaches and their charges can overcome athletic problems and discover athletic solutions. Changing the viewing refers to modifying an athlete's perspective on a problem and creating a mindset that will yield solutions. Changing the doing refers to ways to modify the way a problem plays out so that a static and useless way of performing becomes different and therefore more changeable. By changing the doing the doer is open to alternative ways of performing. Alterations, by definition, create change; change affords the healthiest part of the athlete an opportunity to step through the open door that is then created psychologically.

This chapter will provide several methods for changing both the viewing and the doing of the problem. The methods and techniques that we describe should be imbedded in the hypnotic context. That is, they should be employed after hypnotic induction is complete. They then constitute alternatives for the intervention phase of the hypnotic session. While they are commonly employed outside of hypnosis we believe that they become even more powerful when the hypnotic state is first induced. The interventions then seem to get to an even deeper level of the mind and more easily go into the body. Much of the material that follows has been drawn from the work of Bill O'Hanlon (1989) and that of Insoo Kim Berg (1998) and Steve de Shazer (1988).

# Changing the viewing

## Providing a new frame of reference

When you help the athlete to change his viewing of the situation you're providing him with a new frame of reference. Providing a new frame of reference is useful because it changes perspective and thereby allows for various solutions to be discovered. Sage psychotherapist and teacher, Carl Whitaker, used to say that any time you changed a patient's perspective on a problem you were doing something therapeutic (Neill & Kniskern, 1982). He would sometimes have people view the rest of the family from outside the room through a one-way mirror, or give them an audio- or videotape of the session to listen to or view at the end, so that they could hear themselves and/or see themselves. When you help athletes to change the viewing of the problem by giving them a new frame of reference or perspective you're helping them to get out of the myopic inertia that so often accompanies problematic athletic performance.

Using this method you do as Milton Erickson did, and accept what the athlete states with regard to his perspective and his performance, but then you suggest alternative or different points of views or ways of looking at things. It's important that you validate his original perspective as being the "best choice" that could be made given his experience and his knowledge. Then, in offering alternative perspectives, you give the athlete the opportunity to go beyond his learned limitations.

One example of this process occurred when a basketball player was told by his coach during his high school career that he was a clutch player and that he was expected to take the last shot or shots in any close game. Having been defined by his coach in such a manner, he developed a self-image and a healthy expectation that then became prophetic of how he actually played. The coach intuitively gave a naturalistic and conversational posthypnotic suggestion for success and created a winning expectation in the athlete. This is tantamount to a therapeutic Pygmalion effect in sports.

Another example whereby someone was able to augment his perspective was the golfer Jack Nicklaus, who was known for visualizing the the preferred outcome of each shot or putt before he actually struck the ball. Elite athletes have an uncanny way of doing the things that we are advocating naturally. It is to our advantage as hypnotic sport psychologists to utilize the methods of success that elite athletes employ to the advantage of all the athletes we encounter.

A lot of everyday phrases that are used in sport parlance are designed to change perspective. For example, in October 2002 at her first horse show in a while with the fences set at four foot six inches, the professional equestrian Janet Edgette was told by her coach, George Morris, that she was "just a little bit rusty". This changed Edgette's dejection over a relatively poor round by altering her perspective on it. Rather than make her think that she couldn't do it, it created the notion that it was just a matter of time until her performance improved. She attributed the problem to something that could be overcome, and *would* be overcome with time.

Another example of the phrase "being in a slump": this implies that the athlete has done well in the past and will, at some later point, break *out* of the slump. We saw a perhaps humorous example earlier of how to overcome a feeling of being intimidated by the opposition: "They put their pants on the same way that you do", says the coach. This is designed to create an unshakable visual image that brings them down to earth. Likewise, the saying "When the going gets tough, the tough get going" is designed to change perspective even in advance of the inevitable adversity every player and team must face.

## Using humor

Milton Erickson was the first therapist to legitimize the use of humor in psychotherapy. While earlier therapists, including Freud, would tell jokes to their patients, often for therapeutic effect, no one ever discussed this as an intervention. Erickson, however, acknowledged and legitimized the use of humor both to drive home a point and, importantly, to change perspective on a problem. When you chuckle at something, you have, by necessity, to assume a different distance from and, hence, perspective on the issue at hand. Even the term "lighten up" implies the merits of taking a different perspective.

The value of using humor in sports can be seen on an everyday basis. For example, team clubhouses greatly value having a practical joker on board at all times. Whether these people are putting shaving cream in a ballplayer's cap or heat in their jock strap, they are not just providing entertainment value but with proper timing are keeping the team's intensity level optimal. Likewise, the "rally caps" that baseball players adopt in late innings to create a substantial comeback have the advantage not only of utilizing the expectations inherent in any superstition but also to provide a humorous and even goofy situation that again moderates the intensity level. In tough situations teams can press too hard and try too hard, and, so the tickle of an amusing "rally cap" can get players to loosen up a little and perhaps perform better.

Another example is when you see managers angry about a call that a baseball umpire makes, coming out of the dugout and perhaps ranting and raving or even covering the home plate with dirt in anger. While they seem all too intense, they provide a humorous situation for the team to enjoy. Since this almost always occurs during a downturn in fortunes, this humorous moment, one that almost always results in the manager's being ejected, loosens up a team in a tough situation. Stories like this and/or jokes should be recounted in the body of a hypnotic session.

## Arousing curiosity for athletic success

When an athlete's curiosity is aroused it is most often in order to create a presupposition that something good will happen, and yet the athlete doesn't know exactly *how* it will happen. So curiosity serves to position her psychologically so that she has an anticipation and expectation of success and begins speculating on all the ways that this can happen. Curiosity, then, is a convenient way for us to create a presupposition that success will happen. Curiosity creates an attitude that fosters success in sports.

I (TR) once told the team I was coaching before a state championship game that they had the opportunity in one game, and at one time and place, to achieve all three of their team goals for the year. I reiterated that these team goals were (1) having a winning record, (2) setting a school record for wins, and (3) winning a state championship. At the point that I was saying this the team were nine and nine, and going into a state championship game. The outcome was positive perhaps in part due to my orienting my players to an intriguing and compelling possibility, which then made them curious as to how they could win. The issue of whether they would win was conveniently bypassed by my statement citing the three goals of being attainable in one fell swoop. I had created an assumption that this could happen and then with the team began calculating ways to make the possibility come true. It's important to note that this intervention was done during a team hypnosis session. I also expressed curiosity as to how each player could surprise me and help the team reach their goals.

## Using metaphor and anecdotes

One of the most common ways to change the viewing is to use metaphor and anecdotes. One or more of these can be delivered to the athlete's subconscious mind in the midst of a hypnotic session. Metaphor and anecdotes constitute one major method of intervention in hypnotherapy. The primary way that they accomplish the task of helping the change take place is by altering the athlete's perception or viewing of his situation.

It is important to recognize that the only way the sport psychologist practicing hypnosis can know which metaphor and anecdotes to tell is to have a goal: the hypnotherapist can decide on which metaphor to tell only when she knows to what end the story is being revealed. Knowing the moral or the point of the metaphor or anecdotes allows a proper selection of the information to be revealed.

If, for example, an athlete were dejected and demoralized one might consider telling the story of Lance Armstrong, the cyclist who overcame testicular cancer to return to the peak of his career and win three consecutive Tour de France. It was a 50–50 chance that he would even live, much less compete again. And yet Lance Armstrong credits overcoming cancer with enabling him to appreciate and get the most out of his athletic gifts.

It is best not to leave all your eggs in one basket, though, but instead to tell more than one story to your client. The hypnotherapist might, with the dejected client above, followup the story of Lance Armstrong with a story about the pitcher Roger Clemens, to supplement the hoped-for creation of perseverance with a complementary characteristic determination. Roger Clemens was one of the sport's most dominant pitchers but was thought to be on the decline when the Boston Red Sox traded him to Toronto Blue Jays. This served as a wake-up call to Clemens and he utilized his anger to redouble his training efforts, regain his focus, and win yet another Cy Young Award. Later, when he was traded to the New York Yankees, he found something different to use to improve his performance. He desperately wanted that elusive World Series ring. So again he put himself through an even tougher training regime and got himself his fifth Cy Young Award and more than one World Series ring.

No matter what the psychological goal for a given athlete, metaphor and anecdotes can be assembled from the wealth of colorful and interesting stories that speckle the world of sports. Bear in mind, though, that the one prerequisite to being able to roll out these stories is that you are a fan of various sports. You have to cultivate a broad and general knowledge of different athletes and teams from a variety of sports. It helps to watch many different sports on TV as well as the sports news programs on cable.

That said, once you have a body of stories to choose from, you make your choice knowing the intended goal and it can be as if you were treating your mind as an Internet search engine. That is, prior to your hypnotherapeutic session with a given athlete, you take a contemplative moment, be it in the shower or in the car, and allow yourself to brainstorm, free-associate, meander through your subconscious, so that the key words associated with the intended goal yields some useful stories. While some people can improvise and do this spontaneously, most are better off planning ahead of time which stories and anecdotes they intend to use.

The end result is that depending on the pool of stories that you as an individual hypnotherapist draw from, you might tell one story or another to a given athlete for a given problem. So, for one athlete who has a problem with mechanics on the diving board, the hypnotherapist may tell a story about a pitcher who makes sure that he releases the ball at the same point in his motion by using videotape. Another hypnotherapist might talk about how a golfer, after practicing a particular swing, will "lock it in"—this is an example of "muscle memory". To yet another athlete who loses her focus late in a game, one hypnotherapist may tell a story of track and field sprinters always imagining that the finish line is actually ten yards further away so they don't let up in the last stride, while another hypnotherapist may tell a story of a tennis player who, way ahead in a match, keeps talking to himself about the need to "finish off the opponent".

# Changing the doing

Whereas changing the viewing is designed to alter an athlete's cognition, changing the doing is an intervention designed to modify actions. Athletes who need to alter their outlook should be offered techniques for changing the viewing, whereas athletes who need to alter primarily the enactment of their athletic endeavors on the field or the court can be taught to change the doing.

However, this distinction is somewhat artificial in that many athletes need to have both their viewing *and* their doing altered, but, for the purposes of explanatory clarity, we have separated the two strategies.

## Finding exceptions to the problem

One major way of changing the doing is to help the athlete to reconnect with exceptions to the problem—times when the problem did not happen. These times can be in the present or the past.

Exception finding can be accomplished out of trance, by diagnostic interviewing or in trance by employing the technique of talking in trance (Chapter Six). This can be accessed using the simple command, "Tell me about a time when you were in a very similar situation to the one that you describe, but when things went very well and, not only did the problem not occur, but you were successful". Once an athlete identifies such an exception, the therapist should ask detailed questions about its nuances.

In doing so, the therapist should remember the way in which we were taught to write a news article in high school. That is, remember to ask about the who, what, when, where and why. And, truth be told, the last element, the why, is the least important. Like Milton Erickson, we feel that insight, while it can be personally gratifying, has very little to do with the change process.

So, for example, an athlete age-regressing in hypnosis in an effort to identify an exception would probably happen upon just such an instance. With hypnotherapeutic inquiry using the five Ws of journalism, the subject might discover that the key element that precluded the occurrence of the problem was, for example, a more extensive warm-up that was lately being bypassed.

Finding exceptions is especially helpful in enabling athletes to burst out of a slump. Inasmuch as being in a slump can be defined as the repeated and very frustrating and predictable occurrence of a problem or a situation that endures, scanning the present and the past for exceptions becomes key to ending the slump.

This is the sport psychology equivalent of what so many athletes do anyway in diagnosing the mechanical reasons for any slump. That is, hitters hitting poorly will study extensive videotape of their current stance and swing and then compare that with videotape of when they were hitting well to see what it is that they were not doing back then that they're not doing any longer. Likewise, professional quarterbacks will study clips of successfully completed passes and compare them to clips showing all their interceptions. In this way, they can not only figure out what not to do but can, most importantly, figure out what to do differently.

If an athlete has difficulty identifying a present or a past example of an exception, then she can be encouraged to find an exception in a different area of her life. For example, if she comes to you for a sport psychology consultation related to wanting to have a better work ethic, and then cannot in age regression find a time when she manifested that in her sport, she can be encouraged to find a different place in her life, academically for example, where she did show a very good work ethic. Then the hypnotherapist can encourage the subject, in hypnosis, to disregard the context and content while holding onto the theme or the emotion or the resource and reapplying it to the current athletic context.

## Pattern interruption

Pattern interruption is an alternative to finding the exception in an effort to change the doing. Pattern interruption is a matter of altering the way in which the problem is performed. To accomplish this, hypnotherapists would prescribe in hypnosis the continuance of the problem while suggesting one or more changes in the way in which the problem manifests and rolls out. Milton Erickson believed that, if the way in which a symptom was experienced was altered then the symptom either would not occur or would be more amenable to alteration in therapy. Also, like Milton Erickson, we believe that people are health waiting to happen: the alteration of a symptom or an athletic problem allows the opportunity for health or athletic success to encroach on an otherwise problematic picture. sport psychologist practicing hypnosis can prescribe changes in the pattern of the problem related to the first thing that happens when the problem is experienced; the last thing that happens when the problem is experienced; the time period in which the problem takes place; and, perhaps most importantly, the order or sequence in which the problem unfolds. There are innumerable ways in which patterns can be interrupted. Pattern interruption is a natural part of sport, anyway. For example, coaches try to interrupt patterns of success by the opposition by calling time-outs to ice the field goal kicker or the free-throw shooter. Individuals in sport try to interrupt patterns of success to produce failure in an opponent by, for example, stepping out of the batter's box to interrupt the pitcher's rhythm. Or, conversely, the pitcher will step off the rubber and make the batter wait, so throwing off the batter's timing.

Pattern interruption also occurs naturally in sports in attempts to prevent further failure. For example, a manager might visit a struggling pitcher on the mound, or a basketball coach might call a timeout as a strategy when his team is struggling.

Other examples of pattern interruption to disrupt successful opponents include the infamous temper tantrums of tennis players such as Illie Nastase, Jimmy Connors, and John McEnroe. These players would use their on-court antics and eruptions to throw opponents off balance. But the best players have range and flexibility, and this is greatly needed. It is said that the only reason John McEnroe was able to win Wimbledon over Bjorn "Iceborg" Borg was that he eventually recognized that on-court temper tantrums would be unsuccessful in rattling his opponent, who was known for his unflappable coolness, and would be self-disrupting. McEnroe rose to the occasion and kept a cool head.

The great advantage of hypnosis to sport psychologists is that they can take these time-honored ways in which patterns of failure have been interrupted and disrupted in sport and apply these methods in a focused, intentional, targeted, and intelligent fashion at very deep and enduring levels of the psyche.

## *The miracle question*

While the technique of finding exceptions to the problem requires that the subject go into the recent or distant past through age *regression* in order to identify the exceptions, the miracle question is a procedure developed by Steve de Shazer (1988) that employs the use of age *progression* to discover solutions to problems. To use the miracle question therapists should put their subject into hypnosis and then ask, "If after the session today you were to go about your business for the rest of the day, including eating dinner, and then were to go asleep, if a miracle then happened while you were sleeping, how, upon awakening, would you know it had happened? That is, what would be the first thing that you would notice that would tell you that a miracle had taken place and your sport problem was resolved forever?"

After using talking in trance to hear the answer to this question (although it's important to know that the answer can remain unverbalized and still be effective), such as: the therapist can then ask follow-up questions, such as:

- "Would you be the first person to know that the miracle had happened, or would there be someone else who would have noticed before you?"
- "How would you know that the first other person to notice that the miracle had taken place knew too that it had happened?"
- "How would they know that *you* knew that the miracle had occurred?"

As one structured way of effecting age progression, the miracle question provides a handy methodology for finding solutions. The athlete can use this method, not only with the issue of the moment, but as a tool that she can independently pull out whenever she runs into a problem in her sport. It is a handy supplement to self-hypnosis training.

An example of the miracle question in action might be of an aspiring world-class equestrian who felt as if her riding career was not moving forward at a proper pace. Stumped as to what to do to raise the trajectory of her career, the equestrian went into a self-hypnotic state and asked themselves the miracle question. Upon experiencing the sensation that the miracle had taken place and she was riding at the elite level that she had aspired to, the equestrian performed the "who, what, when, where and why" inquiry and discovered that one of the most important elements of the occurrence of the miracle was the increased use of a trainer to coach both horse and rider. She had been trying to lower expenses by cutting back on those aspects of training in the hopes that she could accomplish the needed training herself without help. Until she asked herself the miracle question, the equestrian was unaware that this approach was what was hampering her.

# Maintenance of the positive changes

Whether through changing the viewing or changing the doing, once positive changes have been made it is useful for the sport hypnotherapist to focus on how to help the athlete maintain those changes. Often, the problems brought to the offices of sport psychologists relate directly not to solving a problem, but more to avoiding falling back into counterproductive ways. So, whether it is ensuring the continuance of a newfound change or precluding a pattern of relapse, an emphasis on maintaining changes is helpful to most athletes. To this end, what can be called *maintenance questions* can be asked of the subject in hypnosis.

Maintenance questions can be, for example, "What do you need to do so that these changes will continue?" or "What is the first thing that you'll notice if you are about to backslide, and, when you notice that, what will you do to preclude losing the change?" or "What process or procedure or ritual can you put into place so that your patterns of success continue uninterrupted?" It is important to note here that rituals are the everyday way in which athletes lock themselves into patterns of success. Whether it's checking shoelaces and then bouncing the basketball a certain number of times before shooting a free throw or stepping out of the batter's box and going through a ritual of swinging and stretching, athletes in every sport have pre-game, intragame and post-game rituals that are not mere superstitions but serve to lock them into their patterns of success.

By asking solution focused maintenance questions and then using talking in trance to honor and acknowledge the answers interpersonally, the sport psychologist is effectively teaching the athlete with a problem something that some, even many, fortunately do effortlessly and naturally. Again, we have an instance where good sport psychology mimics in a thoughtful and targeted fashion what successful athletes do naturally.

# III

## Transcripts of Clinical Sport Hypnosis

# Chapter Nine
# *A Golfer With A Hitch*

There follows a transcript from a session with a golfer, Steve, who was a perfectionist to the point of becoming paralyzed and losing the fluidity of his stroke. His intensity would rise to the point where he would bring his golf club back but be unable to "pull the trigger" and bring it forward.

I (JHE) worked with this client using a vast array of hypnotic techniques, including posthypnotic suggestion, amnesia, positive hallucination, negative hallucination, age regression, and age progression. All of these hypnotic phenomena are deployed to eliminate and indeed preclude the paralysis that would result from the intensity of this client's efforts. For example, the age-regression intervention was used to bring him back to a time period when his stroke was fluid and easy and he would go with the flow. This would have the effect of helping him to "reset" his subconscious mind so that it went back to that time period. Age progression was used to give him an undeniable sense that he could relax and remain fluid in future moments. Both of those interventions create an expectation and a mental stance so that the paralysis resulting from rising intensity is circumvented.

I also used hypnotic techniques to change the experience of the moment, so that the client didn't put pressure on himself. The situation, atmosphere and context are changed through the production of positive and negative hallucinations. Negative hallucinations remove something from the golfing situation; positive hallucinations add something. You'll see that typically what are removed are elements that contribute to the high anxiety and effortfulness, and the elements that are suggested to appear (positive hallucinations) are those that, through the initial interview, were found to create exceptions to the problem, times when the movements needed for golfing were smooth and fluid.

Posthypnotic suggestions, as well as amnesia, are used to alter the client's memory and therefore to alter his habitual reaction of mounting anxiety. Amnesia is first employed to help him to forget situations and anxiety triggers so that the pattern doesn't even begin. Erickson taught that if you could preclude the first element of a pattern from taking place the rest of the pattern would not follow. Posthypnotic suggestion is used to complement amnesia and ensure that what does happen is the first step to success–relaxation and comfort. I'm making an intervention on the same element from two different angles: one approach is to remove what creates the problem; the other approach builds what should be the solution.

Here is what was said to Steve:

People usually go into hypnosis most easily with their eyes closed, and so you can allow yourself to focus on the sound of my voice knowing we're going to… You told me that you're a perfectionist so we're going to

| |
|---|
| *Focusing of attention for induction.* |

begin to modify that right from the get go. Knowing that there's nothing that you need to do here, now, you can rest there and I'll do all of the work. You're going to be amazed at how your subconscious mind can learn and develop this alternative system of control where less is more—more or less—and the harder you try the less you get and the less you try

the more you get. So, as you breathe in and breathe out, you can recognize that that's a natural act and one that you don't need to think about. Your body, Steve, has a wisdom all it's own. So with every breath you take, in and out, you may find that you go one-hundredth deeper into hypnosis. And it's hard to notice a one-hundredth change—it's impossible to notice a change of one per cent.

| |
|---|
| *Confusion, induction, and induction via suggestion for perfectionism.* |

| |
|---|
| *Suggestion for choices to override the conscious mind.* |

And so you're going to need to adopt more of a look-and-wait-and-see attitude and notice it over time and in time as it accumulates. And the progression can be a geometric progression and the amount of relaxation and comfort

you feel can increase geometrically too. Your conscious mind might feel tempted to effortfully make the hypnosis happen. But here and now, just like it will be, there and then, your subconscious mind takes over and your conscious mind relinquishes just like it did a very, very long time ago, when you first learned to float on water, Steve.

And maybe it was in the ocean, the smell of the salt water and the sound of the seagulls up above; the waves gently, on a calm day, lapping. Or maybe it was in a chlorine pool and you could smell the smell of the chlorine and feel the warmth of the sun beating on your skin. And, as you relax more and more, you recognize that every time you try to float on your back, and you try to make your body float, it doesn't work—you sink. And maybe you have to go through that once, twice, three times.

Some people have to go through that four times, five times, six times ... seven times, eight times, nine times, ten times. But sooner or later, ... later ... now sooner, you recognize that if you give up, you get, if you relinquish, you have, if you ... believe that it can happen

| |
|---|
| *Metaphor of floating on water to alleviate effortfulness.* |

and trust in your body, it will happen, because it doesn't make any sense that a heavy physical body can float on something ... like water. Doesn't make any more sense than thinking you can hit a little white dimpled ball hundreds of yards with a metal stick.

But, thankfully, your body knows an awful lot more than *you* know that you know, and your conscious mind can be hereby disabled when you play golf as it once was when you learned to float on water as a boy. . . but it's not a once and done kind of thing. Very often, your mind needs to relearn. You're in the pool; maybe there's a little bit of a wave in it and gets you a little nervous and you try and float and immediately you sink. There's opportunity to learn and relearn both here and there. Eventually, you learn to float on water so that you can sustain it for a longer period of time and not even a wave getting water in your nose would rattle you enough that you would get effortful and sink.

So you learn that you can flow with the glow and grow with the go as you flow ... smoothly, letting the game of golf flow through you. You are a container, a vessel, you are a conduit for the game of golf and

| |
|---|
| *Clang Association used for a confusion induction.* |

your conscious mind doesn't even have to be there. You can be a silent witness to what your body knows how to do. And you don't need to think, just like right now in hypnosis. You notice your conscious mind is becoming quiet. All that mind chatter is diminishing and stopping and you're learning how to be in the moment. This is part of the flow experience that athletes enjoy having; and now you're going to know exactly how to create it for yourself. By remembering the sound of my voice; by remembering the

| |
|---|
| *Posthypnotic suggestions for self-hypnosis.* |

soft cushions and pillows on your back; by remembering the feelings of hypnosis that you have inside.

Every time you pick up the ball and feel the dimples, you can have as much of this sensation of inner peace and quiet as you would like. Every time you grip the club, the first time you take the club, that will be your trigger to have these feelings come back over you so that you can allow yourself to be purer conduit for the game of golf. You're a host for the game of golf ... True golf is not a game of perfection and I don't even think it's a game of confidence. I think it's a game of learning how to trust yourself and relinquish control. Golf is a game of relinquishment. And you notice how easy it is to be in hypnosis because the chatter of the mind, what the Zen Buddhists call monkey mind, drops off and you can focus on the sound of my voice and the things that I say can influence you very deeply, if they're right for you...

| |
|---|
| *Solution focused age regression to an experience of success.* |

Now, I'd like you to go back in time to a different time period. It can be as if you're in a time machine of sorts and you can go to the time when you shot one of those nice low-scoring games prior to taking any of the lessons that got you thinking too much; you don't need to think. Thinking and intensity has served you well in many life endeavors; it does not serve you well when playing golf. You cannot will a good shot: you need to have a silent inner wish for it and then hope and allow your body to execute it accordingly. Effort doesn't help. You mentioned to me earlier today that you've gotten a lot of mileage out of being intense and intent and trying really hard to be perfect. I think it serves you very well as an attorney. I think it serves you well in life.

You can leave those qualities in the trunk of your car when you take your golf bag out; you can put them in. Later, after your game is over, and you put your clubs back in the trunk of your car, you can take back out your intensity, your perfectionism, and you can put it back on for use for the rest of the day. Just as you change your shoes to play golf, you can change your personality to play golf. You can disable certain qualities, you can enable others ... all the while learning to flow with the glow and

| |
|---|
| *Posthypnotic suggestions for a dissociation from a psychological train.* |

| |
|---|
| *Confusion intervention to enable effortlessness.* |

grow with the flow as you row, row, row your boat, gently down the stream, merrily, merrily ... Did you ever have a song that you can't get out of your head? Perhaps that would be useful for you on the course. To keep a certain pace and tempo, to maintain a certain lightness. You can develop certain rituals to keep you associated and locked in, to keep you locked into certain helpful patterns. You can disable and push off to the side certain personality qualities that aren't useful.

Golf's a great way to grow, evolve, and become enlightened. Whatever personal tendencies don't serve you well, you'll learn about them on the course. And now, I'd like you very much, Steve, to immerse yourself. Find yourself playing golf that day when you shot the very low score and you're in the flow and you're letting it happen naturally. You don't need to make it happen: you can let it happen. You trust, trust, Steve, and you can hear the sounds from the day; you can look out and see the course. Feel the tee between the fingers, smell the special smells, feel the slippery soap of the ball wash. And all of these things can create a certain reverie for you. And here you are, shooting a low

> *Age/future progression to the desired performance.*

score. Not even thinking about it, just letting it go, flow through you. And you can memorize this game, this day, this moment, and you can imagine yourself putting a hand up to your brain and pushing a reset button on your brain: you're resetting your inner golfer, so that this becomes the baseline, this is the new learning.

> *Cease-and-desist suggestion.*

You know the subconscious mind is very good at acquiring a learning and then using it all over the place, even where it doesn't belong. Your subconscious mind, with that intensity and perfectionism made for victory but now it needs to back off from putting that into your golf game because that's one place where it doesn't belong. So you can thank your subconscious mind for trying to use the usual methods of your success on the golf course but you say thanks and no thanks. And you know that, and you know what it means to let go of the intensity. You know what it means to let go of the perfec-

> *Hypnotic resource retrieval of a quality already manifest.*

tionism, to be more low-key, easygoing, and relaxed because you do it in your family life. There's not much use for those qualities in family life. So you're already an expert at leaving it out of a certain place in your life, a certain arena. And now you can leave it out of the golfing arena as well. Remember, there's a special place for it to be in the trunk of your car ...

And you mentioned to me how you try too hard at the range and no doubt when you're playing. But you don't try so hard when you're golfing at home and you've got the net in front of you because you don't know where the ball's going to go and you don't know a lot of the particulars, so you just focus on your stroke, making every stroke count. You practice hitting the ball into the net. Now I don't know if it's going to surprise you

> *Age regression to practicing at home, hitting into a net.*

or whether you're going to expect it, but it's going to be as if that net appears on the range, on the course, everywhere. It's going to be as if it just automatically pops up ... wherever you go.

> *Posthypnotic suggestion for experience.*

Maybe you'll imagine it coming out of the ground, popping up. Maybe it'll drop down from the sky. But it pops up. You first take a gander at where you are, what you're shooting for, where you're shooting. But then it pops up and you're not going to want; you have a certain intention in your heart, and then you just swing and you let go of the outcome. There's a wonderful story about this kind of thing in the book *Zen in the Art of Archery* (Herrigel, 1989), where the man learning archery from the Zen masters effortfully tries to hit a bull's-eye, over and over and over again, to no avail. And then they blindfold him and have him feel where the target is. He

> *Metaphor for letting go. Suggestion for negative hallucination and amnesia.*

becomes expert at hitting the bull's-eye even though he's blindfolded. Would it be okay if you blindfolded yourself? You can pretend anything and it will be real. You can allow yourself to experience this as real. And you can forget about the score and you can forget about how you're doing and you can forget about how many shots it took you to get to where you are and yet every shot is the only shot.

You have amnesia for the ones before and you have amnesia for the ones that will be on the next hole. You are anchored in the shot you're making; you make every shot count. You honor the shot, not by trying hard or by being a perfectionist but by bowing to it. That shot's the only shot that exists. At the end of the hole—your score—your amnesia will lift temporarily. Your score will come to you, you can record it, but then it's out of your mind immediately. You don't need to have that awareness; you're better off not being aware. Years ago when Greg Norman was falling apart, I predicted it because I said he's too far ahead; he's going to start to think. He started to think, "Don't blow it!" instead of thinking to himself, "Enjoy!" Forget about the score. It's good to forget about the scores. It's good to forget about what the people you are playing with are doing and you are in the shot and you make every shot count. You give your heart to every shot. It's a sacred pursuit and you go with the flow and flow with the glow and yes, you will grow.

| *More suggestions for age progression.* |
| :---: |

So, with this in mind, I'd like you to hop in that time machine and move forward to the future. And I'd like you to take a couple of moments to allow yourself to project yourself into different scenes. Scenes of golfing situations that you are going to be in in the coming weeks.

Then notice how each and every time you are blindfolded, notice how or each and every time how up pops that net and you can't see the course. You saw it originally. You know where you're shooting for but you are just going to take a stroke. That's right ... and so you're projecting yourself into different scenes. Different

| *Suggestions for positive and negative therapeutic hallucinations.* |
| :---: |

scenarios that you actually step into for a couple of moments while having the mindset that we've cultivated, while having the comfort inside. The silent mind, the conscious mind, is just observing—it's there, it's a witness. Your conscious mind is witnessing the game of golf flow through you. You're a pure vessel containing the conduit. That's right. And you are experiencing this and it's work will be in all those situations and you're trying it on for size; you're getting used to what it's going to be like right now.

| *Posthypnotic suggestions for enabling hypnosis.* |
| :---: |

With this in mind, I would like you to recognize that when you come out of hypnosis, you can keep these feelings and that they will come back to you. All of these suggestions and all of the feelings that you've cultivated inside will come back to you when you pick your clubs out of the trunk, or they'll come back to you when you touch the

ball; and every time you grip the club you'll go into this zone. So, with this in mind, I would like you to allow yourself to take one, two, or three deep breaths and allow yourself to begin to wake up all over, feeling refreshed and rejuvenated, centered and suggestible. Waking up all over.

## Follow-up

The client was contacted six months after this session and gave feedback on the session's effectiveness. "After our last session back in early September," he told us, "I ended up playing golf a week later and another round of golf with a group of folks about two weeks later. Then I had played a few holes around the course, type of thing, in October. Didn't get a chance to play as much as I would have liked for the rest of the fall.

"The last session was a huge, huge help and basically I feel like I am back. It's amazing how enjoyable the game of golf has gotten again. The scoring was better than it had been—certainly not as good as it had been in the past but certainly better than it was with my recent struggles over the last year. The most important thing is just [that] the enjoyment of the game is so much greater now.

"The second round I played in September was with a guy who had been out with a group of us when we played in June and he said that he couldn't believe the difference in my swing and in my game. I want to thank you very, very much. I thought the three sessions built on each other and improved on things we had already done. I am actually looking forward to getting out and playing as the weather gets better. In fact, it looks like I'm going to have the opportunity to play in mid-February out in Palm Springs at a client's annual meeting and I'm looking forward to it. I haven't really had a chance to get back into the tapes again, but I probably will before I play again."

# Chapter Ten
# *Team Hypnosis*

This chapter will discuss the use of hypnotic technique and hypnotic phenomena to enhance athletic performance at the team and individual levels. In the upcoming edited case example, I (TR) apply ideas from the field of hypnosis to a soccer team I coach. I have used similar approaches with my soccer teams for the last eighteen years. Many of my players are convinced this has had a major impact on their performance at both the psychological and neuromuscular levels.

Although I have not emphasized induction and deepening techniques in this example or with my teams, others could easily incorporate both concepts to their specific sports challenges. I was not interested in utilizing induction or deepening techniques with high school students. I knew I could attain desired results without induction and deepening.

Nevertheless, hypnosis can be induced, even deeply, by using hypnotic technique and eliciting hypnotic phenomena.

Another unintended possibility is a double-induction scenario invoked naturally by the format used. This could happen because the hypnotic technique was done within a group setting that also incorporated work at the individual level of performance. This would be an induction within an already established induction. While working on individual goals for their next game, players were invited to "surround" their individual game plan with their team game plan.

The team's game plan evolved from a discussion between the coach and team and was written on the chalkboard. In the case example below, the team's game plan is denoted by headings and italicized script. After the team plan was completed, the players were asked to lie on the floor and the lighting was dimmed. A version of this format was used the day before each game.

The hypnotic techniques and hypnotic phenomena utilized in this case were drawn from the work of Edgette and Edgette (1995), Lankton and Lankton (1983), Erickson and Rossi (1979), Erickson, Rossi and Rossi (1976), and Haley (1973). The techniques and phenomena incorporated include age regression, age progression, resource retrieval, seeding, linking, posthypnotic suggestion, and awakening. A recent innovation used is the concept of "making a correction" drawn from the work of Liggett (2000).

This is how it went:

Take a deep abdominal breath, hold it, hold it, hold it, and exhale. Take another deep abdominal breath, hold it, hold it, hold it, and exhale. From infancy to the present, each of you has mastered a variety of motor skills. As an infant, you are unable to hold up your head, but, with practice and determination, you master that. Moving forward in time, you find it very difficult to even crawl, but you practice and practice and eventually become quite good in crawling, walking, running. And then there came the time when each of you master riding a two-wheel bike. Your little legs pushing down on the pedals, those small hands gripping the handlebars, and the feel of wind on your cheeks as you went faster and faster and felt more and more confident.

*Relaxation, age regression, and resource retrieval.*

Are you practicing with your mother or father? Are there training wheels on your bike? Look down. Are they there or not? The day they come off, I'll bet one of your parents is running down the street with you holding on one way or another. They finally let go and you are able to ride for the first time on your own without any help whatsoever. As you master that motor skill quite nicely, it is just the start of so much more to follow. Is there a big smile on your face showing your sense of pride and accomplishment for a job well done?

*Seeding for mastery of motor skills.*

Then as you got a little bit older, you become interested in sports: soccer, basketball, whatever sport it may be that you like and you practice and practice. Kicking, trapping, heading, and shooting are but a few of the skills you repeat over and over in soccer. You improve day after day until one day you become a soccer player in high school. At your practices you work very hard in the execution of various skills and you improve week after week.

| *Pacing and leading for making a correction.* |
|:---:|

So what I would like you to do today is to work on the correction that we have been talking about. Pick some aspect of the game that you last played that did not turn out the way you would have preferred. In other words, some aspect of the game where you performed in a manner that you do not feel is an accurate indicator of your true athletic capability. It could be trapping, it could be passing, it could be shooting, I really don't know. Allow some ideas to come to mind about how you would have liked to have played differently in your last contest. See yourself playing the way it was and then make the correction in slow motion. Then see yourself playing the way that you would have preferred to have played. Make it multisensory: what it would look like, how it would sound, and how it would feel. Repeat that image in slow motion the way you would like it to have been several times. Then, after you have been able to do that on several occasions, speed up the motion to regular speed and see yourself playing in your preferred style. Of course you know by now we call this neuromuscular training. It all developed from those earlier skills when you learned how to improve motor activity with desire, determination, and hard work.

Next, I would like you to pick some aspect of the game that you would like to be awesome in tomorrow as we work toward our next victory. This will be your individual game plan that we have been working on since the beginning of the season. See yourself playing the way that you would prefer, what it would look like, how it would sound and how it would feel. Experience performing with perfection some aspect or several aspects of the game important to you so

| *Age progression.* |
|:---:|

that you can be the best player on the field in your position for our team as we go for another victory tomorrow. See it as if you are looking out of your own eyes, hear it, and feel it. For example, if we were talking about a chest trap, you watch the ball coming to you in the air, you hear the sound of the ball as it strikes your chest and feel that stinging sensation. The ball then drops down to your foot and you make the pass or the shot.

| *Age progression of team game plan.* |
|:---:|

While you are working on your individual game plan, I will now surround it with our team game plan. Our team game plan for tomorrow will be:

137

## Short passing game

*The short passing game is what fuels our team to victory and what has led us to such a good season so far.*

## Positive communication

*In order for the short passing game to work we need to have positive communication. In other words, find a constructive way to communicate with your teammates that will help to elicit their best performance.*

## Misdirection

*Misdirection will be a part of our game plan where we want to change fields. We want the ball to go from one side of the field to the other so we can catch our opponent in a weak-side deficiency.*

## Ball control

*We want to control the tempo. We can best accomplish this with our short passing game so that we can be in a position to keep the other team from getting the ball.*

## Intensity

*We need to be intense from the beginning of the game.*

## Unity

*We have had team unity and we need to continue it.*

## No dead-ball plays

*We know the danger of a dead-ball play close to the goal when an opponent might be able to score on us.*

## Hustle

*Hustle always is a way to make up a difference.*

## Intimidate fairly and early

*Intimidate fairly and early and go through the ball on all 50/50 plays so that we can establish dominance from the beginning of the game.*

## Maintain your composure

*Maintain your composure at all times so that we can play the way that we prefer.*

## Focus

*We want to be focused and in the zone so that we can do the things the way we want to do them.*

## In the zone

*When in the zone, it is as if nothing else exists but us and the game and whatever it is that we are working on at that moment in time.*

## Head balls

*We want to continue to work on head balls; being able to head the ball to another teammate, to use a head ball when trying to get out of trouble defensively and also to score.*

## Play the whole game and overlapping

*We need to play the whole game and everyone needs to overlap. We need our offensive personnel to come back and help us on defense and vice versa. We need overlapping offensively and defensively with the use of triangles so we can pass efficiently from one player to another.*

## Weak side help on defense

*We need to maintain our diagonals.*

## Transduction

*The concept of transduction, that is, changing from one form to another so for those of you who want to work on more speed and quickness you might pretend, for example, that you are a cheetah. You can be the cheetah and possess its speed and grace. As you attack the weaknesses of your opponent, you sense their vulnerability and that inspires your play. With this surge of adrenaline, you find your speed and quickness increasing effortlessly as you take control and rule the field of play. Also, for those of you who want to come through the ball with more power and without fear of being injured, imagine yourself as a locomotive and how powerful that is as it goes through anything in its path. So you can imagine yourself as a locomotive and going through the ball with power and no fear whatsoever.*

## Crisscross

*We want to make sure we do our crisscross where the strikers go to the wing and the wing comes into the center. If our opponent plays a flat line, we want the ball to go through the seam or over top so we can get in a one-on-one with the keeper.*

## Positive attitude

*A positive attitude, something that we know makes a major difference; combined with heart and getting pumped.*

*More age regression and resource retrieval.*

This will be our game plan that surrounds your individual game plan for tomorrow's victory. Our team game plan will bring out the individual talents of each one of you so that we can establish mastery as well as exploit the weakness of our competition.

Next, I would like you to go back into a time in your life when you were younger and that could have been a year ago, two years ago, six weeks ago, or even earlier, when you felt powerful, in control, and knew you could do anything that you wanted to do. You are in the zone, you have it, you know that you can do it and you are on top of your game, playing your best. You brought your "A" game you are unstoppable and not to be denied. Experience what that looks like, how it sounds and how it feels. Enjoy all the details of this event, who is there, how old are you, what is taking place? Allow the content to fade

*Linking.*

and bring that powerful feeling from the past and link it to your game plan for tomorrow's victory. See yourself, feel yourself and hear yourself playing with even more confidence and power. You are more awesome than even the first time when you worked on your individual game plan.

*More age progression and linking.*

Next, I would like you to project yourself into the future. We have won our game, and what is it that you read about in the paper the next day that you or your teammates did that contributed to our victory? Also, after the game and the next day in school, what did you talk about with your teammates, friends, and parents that contributed to our win? Allow these future memories to come to mind or create future memories and then bring them back to the present and link them to your game plan and see yourself playing even more awesome and more powerful than on the other occasions so far this year.

Last but not least, before you go to sleep tonight, say to yourself, "This is the way that I want to play tomorrow in our victory. While I'm sleeping tonight, I would like you, my unconscious mind, to practice this over and

*Posthypnotic suggestion for hypnotic dreaming.*

over while I am sleeping. Since I dream anyway, these are some of the memories that I want to create in my mind while I am asleep." What would it look like? Give it an image of what it would look like, how it would sound and how it would feel like and tell your mind to repeat that as you dream throughout the evening.

Now the ideas that we have discussed today are seeds that can be grown and made more powerful. We can program our dreams while we are asleep and this can contribute to awakening tomorrow morning with the expectation of success. While talking about the game with your friends and teammates of how it is that you would like to play, a process

*More posthypnotic suggestion for dreaming.*

is initiated. Then when we enter the field of play and start stretching, the seeds that we have sown here today can be made more powerful and they can blossom and put us in a position to be victorious in our next contest.

So take a moment for self-appreciation for a job well done. You are undefeated against area competition. You have had a great season so far and we want that to continue. So everything that we do with our psychological preparation augments momentum toward our next win. The unconscious mind is fertile ground where these ideas can take root and grow.

*Awakening.*

Now count back from five to one and when you get to one you can feel refreshed, alert as if you had a nice peaceful rest while we worked on our game plan both at the individual level and at the team level for our next victory.

## Use with other athletes and sports

With college, adult amateur, or professional athletes, induction and deepening techniques could be discussed and incorporated as part of an overall game plan if the athlete or team so desired. For a different sport, the overall format can be replicated even though the specific content would necessarily be different.

# IV

## *The Business of Sport Psychology*

# Chapter Eleven
# *Marketing Your Sport Psychology Practice*

This chapter will discuss a number of useful ways to build your sport psychology practice. By using these tips, you will, we think, find it surprisingly easy to begin working with athletes and have them appear in your clinical day. It's important to note, though, that few if any private practitioners can have a caseload filled only with athletes. Even sport psychologists employed by professional sport teams almost always have a separate practice or a different position on the side.

Having a specialty in brief clinical sport psychology allows you to diversify your clientele and thus avoid burnout; allows you to have interesting and sometimes famous clients (exciting and rejuvenating in itself); and allows you to have a separate stream of referrals that are outside the managed care pipeline and stranglehold. Readers interested in developing a sport psychology specialty should be prepared to spend at least a couple of hours a week developing their practice and marketing it. As with other specialties, it will take a number of years to develop a significant clientele that replenishes itself as current clients are finished.

## *The time-honored method: word of mouth*

Sport psychology is intriguing. It's also sexy. And, because it's cutting-edge, politically correct, and a rather positive endeavor, you can unabashedly mention at parties and other social occasions that you do it. Whereas it would be rather tacky to mention to a thin woman at a party that you often work with anorexic, and whereas it's really hard to get many referrals by chitchatting with oddly behaving folk in the grocery store to the effect that you work with severely disturbed borderlines, the mere mention of sport psychology often results in your piquing someone's interest, even if that someone is interested on behalf of a friend or a child.

And, with sport psychology, once you get started there's a snow-ball effect and people will do your marketing for you. It is just like the situation with smoking cessation. If you cure a couple of smokers of their habit, they'll boast to everyone in the office and at parties that they've given it up using hypnosis. Where-as few will boast in a similar fashion about having overcome suicidal tendencies using hypnosis, smokers and athletes alike unabashedly and gleefully sing the praises of hypnosis. Far from being stigmatized, athletes often feel proud of what they've done.

So, talk it up!

# *Office materials*

Another marketing ploy is to develop materials for your waiting room that people can take and give to friends and family. Our waiting room has displays that hold numerous articles on sport psychology and it's use by professional and everyday athletes. These educational pieces have our card stapled on the back page. Sometimes they're out on the table; sometimes they are mixed in with the magazines. Often people call us after months or years, having been given that article by someone.

Also in your waiting room and at all times in your briefcase, for distribution whenever needed and whenever possible, should be a classy brochure that describes the services you offer and your credentials. Try to avoid brochures that look too "home-grown" as they will not look "classy" enough and will be unconvincing.

The professional starting out in marketing sport psychology as a part of his or her practice should also invest money in letterheads and cards.

# Yellow Pages

Some may be surprised to know that a Yellow Pages ad or a mere mention of sport psychology tends to do rather well. We say "mention" because as a part of a general practice ad we've had good success using but one line that lists this specialty. Often no one else in a regional phone book has a similar specialty of sport psychology listed. So each month clinicians so inclined often receive a number of calls and a couple of clients from this advertising. We would be willing to bet that your Yellow Pages ad or Yellow Pages mention might be the only one in your area.

# The Internet

Month by month it seems to be more and more common that referrals will come through the Internet. Having your own web-site ensures that people will be able to find you, often from far-off regions. And, if you're willing to do phone consultation, you can serve people from far away. We prefer to have at least one face-to-face meeting if the ongoing work is going to be by phone. However, the Internet does create an opportunity for becoming known in far-flung places.

Often, simply being a good therapist isn't enough to build a full private practice. Practitioners should get in the habit of market-ing to a particular sport. Often this is a sport that the therapist himself plays or played, or perhaps a favorite sport that he's extremely knowledgeable about. The website, of course, can reflect specialization.

Some interesting examples of websites that you can use as a reference include Janet Edgette's equestrian sport psychology page (www.headsupsport.com) and Allen Goldberg's website (www.competitivedge.com).

# Workshops, presentations, and articles

Staying with the theme of marketing to a specific sport, you should devote a significant amount of your marketing efforts to giving free or low-cost talks to local and regional athletic associations. It's also useful to write occasional articles or even a monthly column for newsletters or magazines as an opportunity to get known. This is free advertising and saves a great amount of money over placing display or classified ads.

Giving presentations and workshops for your professional colleagues also helps generate referrals. As is the case with other specialties, your colleagues will see sport psychology not only as something that they do not do, but also as something that does not compete with the services that they offer. Therefore, they will be much more generous in making referrals to you than they might otherwise be if you were looking for clients that they themselves might see. Years ago we developed a highly successful Ericksonian hypnosis practice by writing so many articles and giving so many presentations that, whenever the words "Ericksonian hypnosis" came up, we were the next thought that would come to mind. We've replicated this method with sport psychology and hypnosis.

One more thing about marketing to specific sports and a particular kind of athlete: consider making your choice based on the level of sophistication of the athlete who performs in that sport, while also taking into account the impact that psychological factors have on performance in that sport. That is to say you're going to be more likely to generate clients by marketing to golfers (a sport often played by more intellectually sophisticated and affluent clients who suffer from what their psyche perpetrates on them with almost every shot) than you will be marketing to your local shot putters.

# Sport psychology's marketing mistakes

We have found that a common mistake that people make in marketing their sport psychology services is to take out many display and classified ads. We and others have found this to be an excellent way of spending a lot of money with few results.

Another time-consuming error is to donate a lot of time working for free to high school and college teams in the capacity of sport psychologist. This can be highly gratifying but seldom if ever leads to a paid position or many referrals in years to come. Teams, organizations, and administrators are curious and somewhat grateful, but never seem to suggest a contract and salary after the initial *pro bono* period. It is as if it were somehow taken for granted that it was and will continue to be free of charge, with the end result being that there never seems to be enough money in any of these budgets to fund the position in year two.

# *A word about resources*

At the end of this book we've listed a number of professional organizations, often national sport psychology associations, that have websites and annual conventions. Becoming a part of these organizations and going to the annual conventions allows you to get to know your colleagues and receive referrals from them. Being listed on the organization's directory or its website is also a wonderful way to get a stream of referrals. Web surfers may be skeptical of the shameless self-promotion that you engage in on your website, but sometimes have a much greater degree of confidence in you for your being listed in the directory of a national association.

Two books that we've mentioned previously have excellent material on marketing: *Exploring Sport and Exercise Psychology* (Van Raalte and Brewer, 1996), a useful professional resource anyway, contains a fine chapter on marketing and integrating sport psychology into your clinical practice; and the practical book *Developing Sport Psychology Within Your Clinical Practice*, by Jack Lesyk, is also an outstanding "how-to" book containing a treasure trove of tips on practice in general and marketing in particular—highly recommended.

# Bibliography

DeJong, P. and Kim Berg, I., 1998, *Interviewing for Solutions*, Brooks/Cole Publishing Company, A Division of International Thomson Publishing Inc.

De Shazer, S., 1988, *Clues: Investigating Solutions in Brief Therapy*, W. W. Norton and Company, New York.

Douillard, J., 1994, *Body, Mind and Sport*, Three Rivers Press, New York.

Edgette, J.H. and Edgette, J.S., 1995, *The Handbook of Hypnotic Phenomena in Psychotherapy*, Brunner/Mazel, New York.

Erickson, M.H., Rossi, E.L. and Rossi, S., 1976, *Hypnotic Realities*, Irvington Publishers Ltd, New York.

Erickson, Milton H. and Rossi, E.L., 1979, *Hypnotherapy: An Exploratory Casebook*, Irvington Publishers Inc, New York.

Erickson, Milton H. and Rossi, E.L., 1981, *Experiencing Hypnosis: Therapeutic Approaches to Altered States*, Irvington Publishers Inc, New York.

E.S.P.N., 1999, *SportsCentury: The Fifty Greatest Athletes of the Twentieth Century*, TV programme.

Haley, J., 1973, *Uncommon Therapy: The Psychiatric Techniques of Milton H. Erickson*, Norton, New York.

Herrigel, E., 1989, *Zen in the Art of Archery*, Vintage Books, Washington.

Lankton, S.R. and Lankton, C.H., 1983, *The Answer Within: A Clinical Framework of Ericksonian Hypnotherapy*, Brunner/Mazel, New York.

Lesyk, J.L., 1998, *Developing Sport Psychology Within Your Clinical Practice: A Practical Guide for Mental Health Professionals*, Jossey-Bass, Inc., California.

Liggett, D.R., 2000, *Sport Hypnosis*, Human Kinetics, Europe Ltd, IL.

Morris, G., November 2002, personal correspondence.

Neill, J.R. and Kniskern, D.P., 1982, *From Psyche to System: The Evolving Therapy of Carl Whitaker*, The Guilford Press, New York.

O 'Hanlon, W.H. and Weiner-Davis, M., 1989, *In Search of Solutions: A New Direction in Psychotherapy*, W. W. Norton & Company, New York.

Unestahl, Lars Eric, Edgette, J. and Edgette, J.H., 3–7 December 1986, *Sports Hypnosis*, The Third International Congress on Ericksonian Approaches to Hypnosis and Psychotherapy, Phoenix.

Van Raalte, J.L. and Brewer, B.W., 1996, *Exploring Sport and Exercise Psychology*, American Psychological Association, Washington DC.

# *Resources**

American Psychological Association, Division 47, Sport and Exercise Psychology. 800-374-2721, http://www.psyc.unt.edu/apadiv47.

Association for the Advancement of Applied Sport Psychology (AAASP). 419-372-7233 http://www.aaasponline.org.

North American Society for the Psychology of Sport and Physical Activity (NASPSPA). http://www.naspspa.org.

International Society of Sport Psychology (ISSP), ISWS der Uni BwM, Werner-Heisenberg Weg 39, D-85577 Neubiberg, Germany.

International Society for Sport Psychiatry (ISSP), 316 North Milwaukee Street, Suite 318, Milwaukee, WI 53202. 414-271-2900 http://www.mindbodyand-sports.com/issp.

British Association of Sport and Exercise Sciences (BASES), Chelsea Close, Off Amberley Road, Armley, Leeds, UK, LS12 4HP. Tel/Fax: 0113 289 1020 http://www.bases.org.uk.

**For further information on hypnosis and sport psychology please feel free to e-mail John at johnedgette@cs.com**

---

*Web site addresses were active at the time of going to press.

# Name Index

# Subject Index

## USA *orders to:*
Crown House Publishing
P.O. Box 2223, Williston, VT 05495-2223, USA
Tel: 877-925-1213, Fax: 802-864-7626
www.CHPUS.com

## Canada *orders to:*
Login Brothers Canada, 324 Saulteaux Crescent
Winnipeg, MB, R3J 3T2
or 291 Traders Blvd. E., Mississauga, ON, L4Z 2E5
Phone: 800-665-1148, Fax: 800-665-0103
E-mail: info@www.lb.ca
www.lb.ca

## UK & Rest of World *orders to:*
The Anglo American Book Company Ltd.
Crown Buildings, Bancyfelin, Carmarthen, Wales SA33 5ND
Tel: +44 (0)1267 211880/211886, Fax: +44 (0)1267 211882
E-mail: books@anglo-american.co.uk
www.anglo-american.co.uk

## Australasia *orders to:*
Footprint Books Pty Ltd.
Unit 4/92A Mona Vale Road, Mona Vale NSW 2103, Australia
Tel: +61 (0) 2 9997 3973, Fax: +61 (0) 2 9997 3185
E-mail: info@footprint.com.au
www.footprint.com.au

## Singapore *orders to:*
Publishers Marketing Services Pte Ltd.
10-C Jalan Ampas #07-01
Ho Seng Lee Flatted Warehouse, Singapore 329513
Tel: +65 6256 5166, Fax: +65 6253 0008
E-mail: info@pms.com.sg
www.pms.com.sg

## Malaysia *orders to:*
Publishers Marketing Services Pte Ltd
509 Block E, Phileo Damansara, Jalan 16/11,
46350 Petaling Jaya, Selangor, Malaysia
Tel: 03 7553588, Fax: 03 7553017
E-mail: pmsmal@po.jaring.my

## South Africa *orders to:*
Everybody's Books
Box 201321 Durban North 401, 1 Highdale Road,
25 Glen Park, Glen Anil 4051, KwaZulu NATAL, South Africa
Tel: +27 (0) 31 569 2229, Fax: +27 (0) 31 569 2234
E-mail: ebbooks@iafrica.com